Physician: Time to Invest in Yourself!

WORK-LIFE BALANCE, THE NEEDS OF THE PATIENT, AND MEDICAL-LEGAL RISK MANAGEMENT

Timothy E. Paterick, MD, JD, MBA
Elizabeth P. Ngo, MD

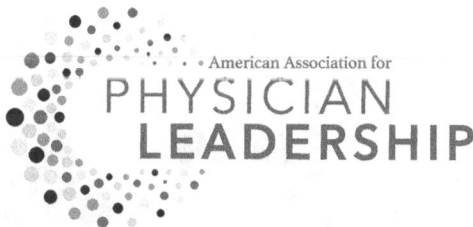

American Association for
PHYSICIAN
LEADERSHIP

13   8 7 6 5 4 3 2 1

Copyedited, typeset, indexed, and printed in the United States of America

PUBLISHER

Nancy Collins

EDITORIAL ASSISTANT

Jennifer Weiss

DESIGN & LAYOUT

Carter Publishing Studio

COPYEDITOR

Pat George

Table of Contents

About the Authors

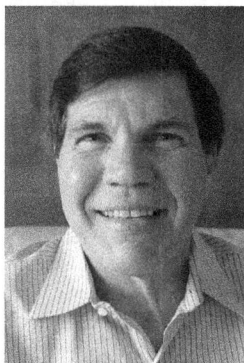

Timothy E. Paterick MD, JD, MBA is a practicing cardiologist with a passion for preventive health measures, sports medicine, and teaching residents and fellows medicine and young people basketball. He trained in internal medicine and cardiology at the Mayo Clinic in Rochester, Minnesota.

Dr. Paterick is a lifelong scholar-athlete. He was named to the top 24 high school basketball players in America his senior year in high school, then matriculated to the University of Wisconsin-Madison on a basketball scholarship. At the University of Wisconsin he was awarded the Ivy Williamson award for outstanding achievement in athletics and academics. After completing medical education at Rush Medical College and his medical training at the Mayo Clinic, Dr. Paterick completed his law degree at the University of Wisconsin followed by his MBA at Edgewood College.

While practicing full-time cardiology Dr. Paterick has written over one hundred peer reviewed articles in the medical literature, has been an invited speaker across the country on medical and legal issues, and authored two books: *Invest in Yourself: A Cardiologist's Narrative for Heart Health* and *Health through Hope: Look in People's Eyes.*

Dr. Paterick's passion is teaching cardiology fellows and young basketball players. Many cardiology fellows, including his co-author, Elizabeth Ngo, MD, have achieved high levels of clinical expertise through his teaching and mentorship. Both his sons, having played Division 1 college basketball, exemplify his basketball-teaching prowess. He attributes any success he has experienced in life to his wife and life-long best friend, Barb. Dr. Paterick can be reached at tpaterick@gmail.com.

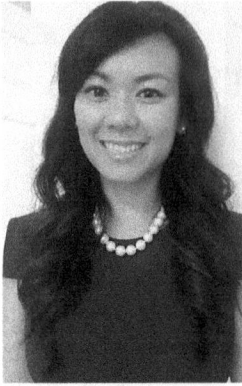

Elizabeth Ngo, MD is a practicing cardiologist whose interests are cardiac prevention and advanced cardiovascular disease. A first generation immigrant, Dr. Ngo has experienced firsthand the cultural, psychological, and financial struggles of coming to a new country and starting from an insolvent background. Through hard work and resilience against odds, she earned a full scholarship to college and graduated summa cum laude which academically and financially paved the road for medical school. The decision to pursue the medical field stemmed from her inquisitive nature to not only understand the complexities of the human body but also the intricacies of the healthcare infrastructure.

Dr. Ngo's varied background makes her a well-rounded, versatile physician—someone who truly understands the multifaceted levels of healthcare from the economic difficulties patients face when seeking medical help to the everyday challenges physicians face in trying to meet the standards of their patients as well as administrators. From her personal and professional experiences, she has become an advocate for self-empowerment through knowledge for her patients, physicians-in-training, and colleagues in hopes of defining a new patient-physician relationship in the modern era. It was during her fellowship that she would meet her mentor, co-author, and friend—Tim Paterick—who not only shared her ideology but encouraged it.

Her facile capabilities not only encompasses perceptive medical knowledge and analytical skills but extends to the aesthetic arena. Dr. Ngo expresses her creative aptitude through writing and visual arts. In her free time, she likes to spend time with her family and husband who have all been an incredible support system for the journey of life. She is an avid runner and enjoys exploring nature and various cultures during her travels. Dr. Ngo can be reached at: elizabethptngo@gmail.com.

Dedications and Acknowledgements

Tim Paterick

Team Paterick: Barb, TJ, and Zachary

My mother and father

Dr. A Jamil Tajik—my teacher, mentor, and friend

Dr. Krishnaswamy Chandrasekaran—
my teacher, mentor, and friend

Dr. Thomas Scott Cunningham—my teacher, mentor, and friend

I want to thank Kate Mannix for her editing expertise.

Elizabeth Ngo

To my husband for keeping my life interesting.

To my family for keeping me grounded.

To my mentor and friend for always inspiring me.

To future and current physicians, may we find a
way to reclaim our profession together.

The Purpose of the Book

"**I**nvest in yourself." That was the message the speaker delivered to the brilliant young students at the University of Michigan business school. They possessed the potential to be innovative, creative, and make a mark in the world. Why would they want to work for someone else? The speaker's message applies to the world of medical professionals as well. Physicians and non-physician clinicians are bright young people who have the potential to change the healthcare landscape and the health of America. That concept became the seed for this book.

Talk with healthcare practitioners and you likely will hear about their discontent with the present corporate healthcare system. This unhappiness can lead to burnout or it can be the stimulus to evoke change that benefits both patients and healthcare professionals (HCPs).

The purpose of this book is to encourage readers to take the time to invest in their own well-being, to become stronger people, so they can lead and advocate for the much-needed changes in the current landscape of medicine. Patient care must always be our number one focus.

The tools and experiences we share here are meant to provide emerging healthcare practitioners with a detailed overview of what to expect along the journey so they can make more informed decisions in building a strong foundation academically, psychologically, and physically. For practicing healthcare providers, this book is meant to help them cope with current challenges they may be facing, whether it's burnout, a medical-legal problem, or the current state of the medical profession.

Physicians and their colleagues must take charge of the health of America. Reclaiming healthcare by physicians and non-physician clinicians (NPCs) will require unification and cooperation. Unification and cooperation will allow physicians and NPCs to sit across the table from corporate entities and arbitrate for the benefit of patients. Motivated by the appeals of autonomy and the commitment to do the right thing for our patients, this

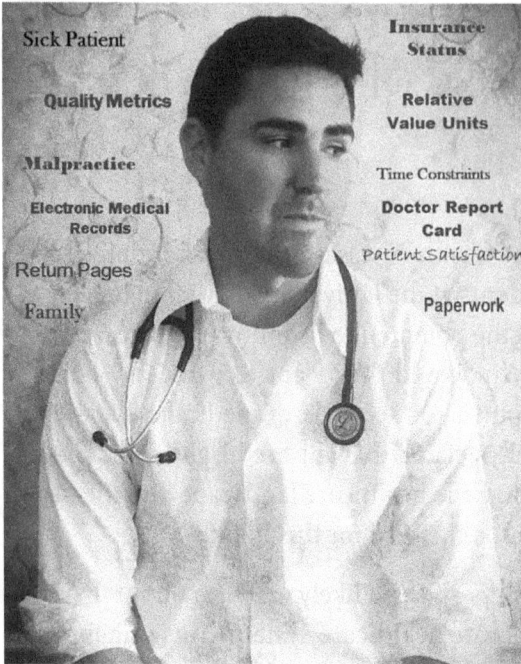

Sick Patient
Quality Metrics
Malpractice
Electronic Medical Records
Return Pages
Family

Insurance Status
Relative Value Units
Time Constraints
Doctor Report Card
Patient Satisfaction
Paperwork

Figure 1.

overwhelming but mandatory unification will allow us to preserve our purpose, save our professionalism, and be fiduciaries to our patients.

Physicians are living in digital time. Their rhythms are rushed, rapid fire, and relentless. Their days are carved into bits and bytes. Physicians practice breadth rather than depth, quick reactions rather than considered reflections. Their actions and activities often skim the surface, lighting for brief moments at multiple destinations. They race from patient to patient and procedure to procedure without time to pause and reflect. They are wired up, but melting down physically and emotionally. Figure 1 gives you a snapshot of today's healthcare provider.

Stop and think about the reality of corporate, balance sheet medicine. It has no true benefits for healthcare providers or patients. The present-day healthcare models are breaking the healthcare bank of Medicare. The healthcare corporations and insurance companies like the model because they are getting cash fat.

Figure 2 graphically identifies the changes we have been experiencing as our country gets sicker and corporate healthcare gets wealthier.

Spend some time studying this graph—it is the embodiment of the saying, "A picture is worth a thousand words." Imagine if we could take all that wasted administrator salary and invest it into patient care. The savings gained by eliminating unnecessary administrators could be reinvested into the health of the public. We need programs on prevention and health maintenance that start in grade school and continue to the residents of assisted

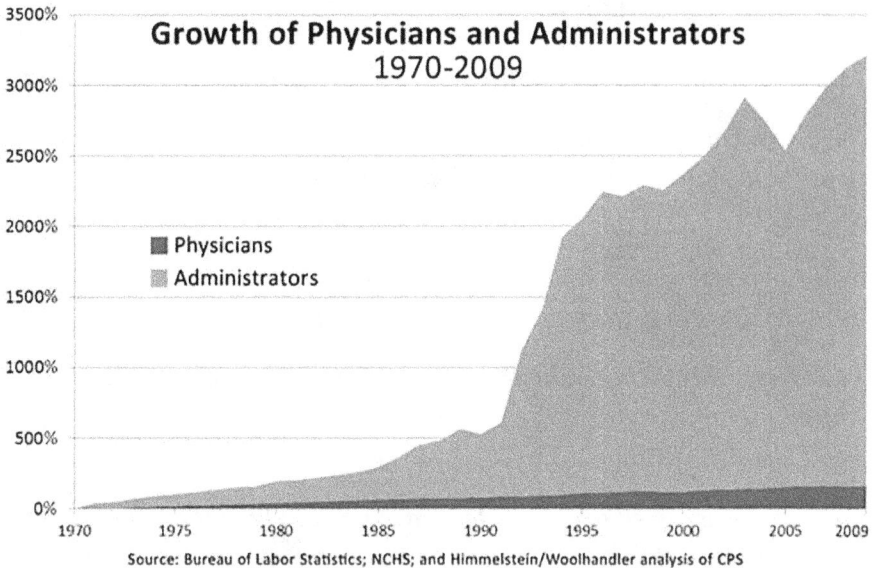

Growth of Physicians and Administrators 1970-2009

Physicians
Administrators

Source: Bureau of Labor Statistics; NCHS; and Himmelstein/Woolhandler analysis of CPS

Figure 2.

living and nursing homes. These programs would reduce health costs and improve the health, vitality, and emotional well-being of all citizens. It sounds simple, but remember that most genius is founded in simple ideas.

We hope this book motivates you to take action for your own well being. We also hope you will unite with other healthcare providers to reach for solutions that give NPCs and physicians autonomy and allow optimal medical education and treatment for all of our society. We cannot ignore the fact that the present-day medical corporate structure is failing the community and the healthcare providers.

HIPPOCRATIC OATH

I swear to fulfill, to the best of my ability and judgment, this covenant:

I will respect the hard-won scientific gains of those physicians in whose steps I walk, and gladly share such knowledge as is mine with those who are to follow.

I will apply, for the benefit of the sick, all measures which are required, avoiding those twin traps of overtreatment and therapeutic nihilism.

I will remember that there is art to medicine as well as science, and that warmth, sympathy, and understanding may outweigh the surgeon's knife or the chemist's drug.

I will not be ashamed to say "I know not," nor will I fail to call in my colleagues when the skills of another are needed for a patient's recovery.

I will respect the privacy of my patients, for their problems are not disclosed to me that the world may know. Most especially must I tread with care in matters of life and death. If it is given me to save a life, all thanks. But it may also be within my power to take a life; this awesome responsibility must be faced with great humbleness and awareness of my own frailty. Above all, I must not play at God.

I will remember that I do not treat a fever chart, a cancerous growth, but a sick human being, whose illness may affect the person's family and economic stability. My responsibility includes these related problems, if I am to care adequately for the sick.

I will prevent disease whenever I can, for prevention is preferable to cure.

I will remember that I remain a member of society, with special obligations to all my fellow human beings, those sound of mind and body as well as the infirm.

If I do not violate this oath, may I enjoy life and art, respected while I live and remembered with affection thereafter. May I always act so as to preserve the finest traditions of my calling and may I long experience the joy of healing those who seek my help.

Introduction

To our future healthcare providers,

Your decision to pursue a career in medicine is an exciting one filled with the anticipation of restoring patients' health, being autonomous, and establishing financial security. The journey to become a healthcare provider can be rewarding academically and personally. However, the journey is arduous; it takes a certain amount of mental fortitude and discipline in medical school to put in the study time required to master the fundamental knowledge that is the foundation of a good physician. Just when you've felt accomplishment in graduating medical school, your physical, mental, and emotional strength will be tested during residency training. Often, during difficult times in schooling and especially during residency or fellowships, students and trainees find themselves asking the following questions:

"How do I make time for myself and my family and friends with all this study and work we have to do?"

"How can I stay ahead of the game?"

"Did I make the right decision to become a doctor??"

To our current practicing healthcare providers,

You've made it through the countless hours of training and now you're a bona fide independent doctor! That sense of elation is quickly replaced by consternation as you now realize you have a whole new subset of challenges to deal with: the business aspects of medicine. Productivity, RVUs, and insurance issues suddenly come into play. Many of you become burned out by the mountains of paperwork that seem to overtake your to-do list.

Add the medico-legal aspect with which many practicing physicians are plagued and yet have little understanding. Questions physicians often ask during this part of the journey include:

"How do I protect myself legally while making the best decisions possible for patients?"

"What should I expect if I become involved in a lawsuit?"

"Did I make the right decision to become a doctor?"

We have been through this experience; we understand the positive aspects of the medical field as well as its tribulations. Hence, this book will provide a roadmap that you can use during your journey to becoming a physician or healthcare provider.

In **Part One**, we provide you with basic tools for achieving a more balanced life and positive experience during your journey in medical school and training. The tools in our toolkit help you handle any challenge with a rational, logical, and systematic approach. We teach you about making the wisest possible investment of your time and energy in order to operate at the highest possible level. We each offer our own perspective on the tools and how we used them.

In **Part Two and Part Three**, we break down the individual components of medical school and residency and present them, again, from two perspectives, each representing a different phase of medical education and training. This juxtaposition is meant to provide you with a panoramic view of medical training—both past and present—and the evolutionary changes that formed the challenges you may face in today's training—in particular the transformation to medical commercialism. We discuss the chaotic medical world physicians' encounter, including the risks of practice and how you can meet the challenges presented to your professional and personal life.

Part Four tackles the present day state of health care and the future challenges.

Part Five is a detailed discussion of medicine and law may intersect, and how it affects physicians and their families.

We hope to provide a comprehensive understanding of the steps involved in becoming a healthcare provider and what a career in medicine means today in an atmosphere dominated by corporate medicine. Although the book is intended as a reference source no matter at what point in the medical journey you are—student, trainee, or practicing healthcare provider—we encourage you to browse the entire scope of the book. As a student or trainee, reading ahead can provide you with insight as to what to expect for the future. As a practicing physician perhaps revisiting the "tool kit" can help you find a way to restore balance and meaning to your life if you are feeling burned out or frustrated.

Your overall goal should be to learn to function by design and not by default. You must drive and control every day of your journey. If you don't design your day, someone else will design it for you. We hope our insight will show you a way to maintain optimum learning, health, and harmony with loved ones, while trekking through the journey of medical education and practice. You will learn how to invest in yourself and your future.

Yours,

TIM AND ELIZABETH

Part One:

The Toolkit

CHAPTER 1

Essentialism

*"Live lives true to yourself instead
of the one others expect."*

—Greg McKeown, author of *Essentialism:
The Disciplined Pursuit of Less*

— TIM'S THOUGHTS —

I strongly recommend becoming an essentialist and living an essentialist lifestyle before entering your education and training.

What is an essentialist? What is an essentialist lifestyle? Essentialism focuses on identifying the important signals in life and eliminating the noise. The noises are the distractions that add no value to your life and frequently monopolize time and meaning. When you assume the role of an essentialist you will discover that you achieve more with less. You will live by design, not by default. This means living proactively rather than reactively. You will systematically and deliberately distinguish the vital signals from the trivial, meaningless noise, and remove obstacles so you can pursue the important signals in a clear, enlightened, and effortless pathway. *Essentialism is a disciplined, purposeful approach that allows you to determine what is important to you and your personal goals, and the best way to achieve these objectives.*

Why is it important to become an essentialist if you are pursuing a life in medicine? Let's answer that question in the alternative by viewing the polar opposite approach: being undisciplined and reactive. The undisciplined and reactive lifestyle leads to you think you can do it all because everything is important. However, ask yourself these two questions:

1. Can you do it all?
2. Is everything important?

The answer to both questions is no. An undisciplined and reactive lifestyle leads you to react impulsively to whatever issue is most pressing at the moment. You say *yes* to all queries without critical thought and execute tasks at the last minute, unprepared. You take on too much and your work product is suboptimal. You feel out of control and become overwhelmed and exhausted. If you do not prioritize your life, those around you will—at the expense of your own energy, time, and personal growth.

How does this apply to you, the evolving healthcare professional (HCP)? As an emerging HCP, you will be challenged to explore, absorb, and learn a vast array of detailed material across a diverse landscape of topics, such as human anatomy, histology, physiology, biochemistry, and pathophysiology. Each topic is akin to a new language that will take time, energy, and cognitive focus to master. This vast amount of material will be set against a background of maintaining your friendships, your family ties, and your health.

How does this apply to you, the HCP? Your work schedule will be dictated by the program or specialty in which you are training. Your work hours will increase exponentially and you will be challenged to fit in continuing education and independent learning as well as a personal life. Many of you will look back, wistful for those "care-free" days of youth. With the current system of healthcare, you will be expected to see more patients, spend time with each patient to accurately diagnose and manage his or her ailments, and complete copious amounts of electronic paperwork to fulfill the requirements of patient and system demands.

A haphazard approach will not suffice when you attempt to meet all these varied demands. Handling this array of responsibilities with limited time will require a well-defined, systematic strategy to use your time, energy, and available resources efficiently and effectively.

ELIMINATING THE NOISE

You must recognize there is an abundance of noise and few things that are exceptionally valuable. You must take the time to explore what is valuable to meeting the demands of school, work, family, and friends. This means recognizing you can't have it all and that you must prioritize. Understanding the reality of these trade-offs will allow you to pursue the priorities that are deemed essential to your survival no matter your stage in life. Spend the necessary time to explore, listen, debate, question, and think about how you will identify the signals among the deafening noise. This detailed and essential exploration will separate the vital from the trivial. You have time and energy only for the vital components of your essential life.

Eliminating noise can be challenging, especially when it has been present throughout your life. You have been meeting everyone's demands for years. Given your new time constraints, that is no longer possible. Saying *no* is difficult. It takes courage. It goes against the grain of all our present-day social norms. Most of us instinctively want to please family, friends, and even colleagues. So it takes mental fortitude and emotional discipline to say *no* to what is socially expected. We must choose what direction to go when confronting noise, or we will be pulled in directions we do not want to go, losing time, and physical and emotional energy on our aimless journeys.

SETTING BOUNDARIES

A key component of essentialism is *boundaries*. These boundaries are constraints that allow you to seek a rich and productive life. Remember, you cannot possibly cope with doing everything for everybody. Despite the mantra spread by the marketing experts, you cannot have it all—and that's okay. The boundaries you establish will protect your personal, emotional, and mental space and time from being monopolized by others. They will prevent you from having to say *no* to people who want to enhance their objectives at the expense of your time and energy. They will allow you to eliminate the demands and encumbrances of others that will not only frustrate you but detract you from achieving your own defined essential objectives and goals. They will allow you the time to explore ways to maximize the use of your time and energy toward what you deem to be important. The boundaries you define are actually liberating and empowering.

TRADE-OFFS

To underscore the necessity of essentialism, let's explore the reality of trade-offs. In the perfect world, we can have all the options in life we desire. Realistically, we often are faced with two choices we really want, but choosing one results in cognitive conflict with the other. For example, you want all As in your didactic work, yet you want more leisure time. Typically there are few times we can have both the grades and the leisure time. This underlies the principle of trade-offs.

Although having to make a choice between two covetable options may be unpleasant, it may also represent a huge opportunity. How? By forcing us to explore and weigh the options systematically and strategically to select the one that will give us the best chance of achieving the desired outcome. Trade-offs should be embraced to make choices deliberately, strategically, and thoughtfully. These deliberate choices create time and space to think and identify what really matters. You may decide to be okay with Bs in exchange for more leisure time. The process of trade-offs allows you to experience addition through subtraction.

In summary, it is important to establish boundaries and utilize trade-offs as opportunities to clarify these boundaries if you haven't already done so. This cognitive process leads to clarity and control of your journey—your journey. This essentialist lifestyle will allow you to enjoy your education and training, as well as your family and friends.

— ELIZABETH'S THOUGHTS —

Essentialism, from a cursory analysis, seems like a selfish lifestyle in conflict with the altruistic principles assumed to be inherent in a career path involving the care of others. Prior to learning about the breadth of essentialism, I followed a few maxims, such as:

- Know your own limitations.
- Everything in moderation.
- Logic goes a long way.

On closer inspection of the concepts of essentialism, I realized it has the components listed above, but is a more succinct philosophy that further delineates the excessive clutter that must be eliminated to streamline your life.

By trying to be a little bit of everything and pleasing as many people in my life as possible, I quickly burned out, suffering from physical, emotional, and mental exhaustion. Ironically, I saw the same weary expression in the faces of colleagues, as well as caregivers of my chronically ill patients, and I advised them to *"Please go home and take care of yourself, because you can only give others optimal care if you're not sick or physically or emotionally drained yourself."* I preached but did not practice this, and in the end, had to deal with the consequences.

In fact, essentialism does not equate to selfishness. Essentialism does not mean putting yourself first among all others at all times. It does not mean being inconsiderate of others around you, nor does it mean carrying out a life of such complete practicality that you lose sight of sentimentality. Essentialism, when practiced appropriately, is a manner of life that allows you to become a stronger and more efficient person—physically, emotionally, and mentally—so you *can* be there for the important people in your life while achieving your own personal goals.

Let's be realistic: As much as we would like to say our happiness is derived solely from helping others, we are human and have our own personal needs and desires. We would be doing a disservice to ourselves and others around us if we were in a perpetual state of denial about this reality. As contradictory as it sounds, you have to be a little selfish in order to be the optimal giver.

For example, after doing a 24-hour shift on call during one Christmas, I was tired beyond words. I wanted to take a long nap and show up just before Christmas dinner, but I knew my family was waiting for me to come early and help prepare the holiday meal. Not wanting to disappoint them, I showed up early to help. However, due to my extreme fatigue, I was disengaged and ended up falling asleep on the couch shortly after dinner rather than participating in the traditional family games. My mom told me she simply was happy to see me and did not expect anything else. It actually made her sad to see me so withdrawn and weary and caused her to worry about me. I should have been "selfish," taken my nap, and shown up to the gathering a much more refreshed, engaged, and cheerful person.

Personally, I think the toughest mental hurdles when embarking on the practice of essentialism are learning to 1) accept that you cannot please everyone and 2) to be a little selfish to be more generous with your time and energy. Many people who enter into the healthcare field have a genuine sense of giving and a desire to please others. They probably will find the above-stated notions difficult to implement. However, once you accept the above concepts, establish boundaries, and prioritize, you can start to experience more balance and peace in your life, which leads to enhanced performance in your service to your patients, family, and friends.

CHAPTER 2

The Necessary Intelligences

"I.Q. is a threshold competence. You need it, but it doesn't make you a star. Emotional intelligence can."

—Warren Bennis, pioneer in leadership studies

— TIM'S THOUGHTS —

The importance of emotional and social intelligence for achieving success in school, career, and in life cannot be overemphasized. Your social and emotional intelligence will prove to be more important than your academic intelligence. We have seen people with high academic aptitude fail in medical training because of poor social and/or emotional intelligence, and people with average academic intelligence, but superior social and emotional understanding, prosper in their medical or surgical training years. Let's look at emotional intelligence and social intelligence and how they play out in the field of medicine.

Emotional intelligence (EI) is the capacity to recognize our own feelings and the feelings of others, understand how these feeling intersect, regulate our feelings, and use this capacity to guide thought and action. EI involves the components of self-awareness, self-regulation, self-motivation, empathy, and social skills.

High EI requires knowing one's self and one's abilities. You must first evaluate your own emotional capacity, make a realistic appraisal of your abilities, and develop a grounded sense of self-confidence. You must then learn self-control, which involves harnessing your emotions in a constructive manner and delaying personal gratification to pursue a higher goal. Once you become aware of your own emotions, you must acknowledge and accept others' feelings (empathy), understand their perspective, and cultivate a dialog in order to reach understanding.

Social intelligence (SI) is the capacity to effectively negotiate complex social relationships and environments. Psychologist Nicholas Humphrey believes that it is social intelligence, rather than quantitative intelligence, that defines humans. Social scientist Ross Honeywell believes social intelligence is an aggregated measure of self- and social-awareness, evolved social beliefs and attitudes, and a capacity and appetite to manage complex social change.

SI, equivalent to interpersonal intelligence, is a person's ability to understand and react appropriately to his or her environment. Neuroscience teaches us that the brain has a large supply of neurons that mimic what another human being is doing. This is our neural Wi-Fi—we detect someone else's emotions through their actions and our "mirror neurons" produce similar emotions within our consciousness. This is identified as the collectively shared experience. Think about the times you feel the happiness of a friend and that resonates so deeply within your being that you feel happy.

Mirror neurons are particularly important for healthcare team (HCT) leaders. Leaders' emotions and actions prompt followers to mirror those feelings and actions. A leader who laughs and elicits positive emotions puts those neurons to work and triggers a spontaneous connectedness and a closely knit team. Being in a good mood helps people take in information effectively and respond nimbly and creatively.

Neuroscience also has taught us about spindle cells. These large cells allow for easy and rapid transmission of thoughts and feelings. The ultrafast connection of emotions, beliefs, and judgments across spindle cells creates what behavioral scientists call our social guidance system. Good leaders, through mirror and spindle cells, are able to connect and resonate with team members, resulting in increased productivity and harmony.

SI is critical in crisis situations. HTC leaders must be able to read the emotional state of nurses and paraprofessional workers to facilitate understanding, empathy, and productivity, and combat the constant changes and vicious cycles of despair in the current healthcare system. We must prevent burnout, a state of mental and physical exhaustion, depersonalization, and a sense of reduced personal self-worth.

There is a large gap between socially intelligent leaders and socially inept ones. Through the course of your training and profession, you will encounter both types of leaders. Our experience suggests that most leaders are intellectually bright, but socially inept. While you are in training, your interactions with the ward clerk, nurses, PAs, NPs, and physicians can be precarious if you are socially inept. Remember that everyone in the work environment is appraising your behavior and judging your character. How they interpret you and who they report to can make or break you. You must be socially and emotionally competent. This is especially important when it comes to choosing your place of employment, since you must know if the leaders there have developed the same subset of skills. That can be a daunting task.

The only way to develop your own social circuitry is to take the challenge of altering your behavior—to rapidly expand your mirror and spindle neurons to allow for exponential humanistic growth. Study people who have developed their social skills. Observe how they read the varying circumstances and how they engage their mirror and spindle cells: the broad smile, the deserved compliment, and even a critique that leads to a motivated team member rather than team despair.

— ELIZABETH'S THOUGHTS —

As important as social and emotional intelligence are, they are not skills that are implicitly taught. Instead, they are acquired through observation of good examples set in the home environment, religious gatherings, or the workplace.

If like me, you grew up in a cultural background where emotional restraint is encouraged and practiced, you may be at a disadvantage when you embark on the professional pathway. Growing up in an environment where you are expected to "tough it out" and "keep it in," there is not much in way of discussions about emotions, let alone teachings or examples.

While emotional evolution was downplayed, didactic knowledge was highly encouraged in my parent's household. Subsequently, my siblings and I did well with schoolwork and eventually acquired the jobs or positions to which we had aspired. However, during a candid discussion with my siblings one day, we realized that while our parents did a great job instilling scholastic skills, we were lacking in social and emotional proficiency, which we realized had a major impact on promotions in the workplace.

This did not mean they were bad parents. In fact, they were incredible people whose sacrifices and generosity led us to where we all are today from an immigrant background: my siblings are engineers and I'm a physician. They basically carried on the cultural idea of emotional suppression they had observed from their parents, and were unaware of the caliber of importance of EI and SI.

Whatever your cultural or environmental background, lack of social or emotional intelligence should not become a default for you. Like academic intelligence, social and emotional intelligence can be learned. Also like academia, it is an active process that requires constant study and practice in order to excel at it. As a matter of fact, Daniel Goleman, a Harvard psychologist, nicely summarized this concept in his book, *Emotional Intelligence*, and coined the term emotional quotient (EQ). Having EQ is not mutually exclusive of IQ. Unlike IQ, which can be established and set genetically, EQ and SI skills are much more flexible and can be learned, implemented, and improved at any age.

If you are entering the medical field, attaining some level of EQ is essential, since it encompasses the component of empathy, which is a skillset most healthcare schools try to imprint on their students. You can start by simply picking a person in your life—coworker, attending, or friend—whose emotional and social intelligence you and others admire, observe his or her actions and reactions to others, and try to learn from these life lessons. Take the time to invest in the improvement of these important intelligences. This ability to understand the emotional well-being of others, empathize, and respond to others will not only be invaluable to your personal relationships, be it a family member or significant other, but in your professional career to communicate, work as a team, and be a leader. As they say, "IQ gets you hired. EQ gets you promoted."

CHAPTER 3

Eat Right, Exercise, Rest, and Play

"Eat to nourish your body. Exercise to be fit, not skinny. Ignore the haters and unhealthy examples. You are worth more than you realize."

Unknown

— TIM'S THOUGHTS —

Advances in healthcare have paved the way to the early identification of cancers as well as genetic and metabolic diseases. Early detection provides an opportunity to practice preventative and sometimes curative therapies in the management of these diseases. Breakthroughs in the evaluation of proteomics and genomics will make this process even easier. Innovations in pharmacology and invasive as well as surgical interventions have been integral in the treatment of many diseases and prolongation of life.

However, despite these advances, there continues to be an epidemic of disease related to unhealthy lifestyle habits that no amount of drugs, surgeries, or medical procedures will cure. An epidemic that is rampant in millions of people. The #1 killer in America is coronary artery disease (CAD), which is a disease of lifestyle choices.

We now know the pathophysiologic process involved in the development of atherosclerosis. Inflammation plays a key role. The risk factors for inflammation and progression of atherosclerosis include hypertension, smoking, diabetes, obesity, Omega-6 overload, Omega-3 deficiency, excess trans-fats, and emotional stress. These are all risk factors you will implore patients to combat—but don't forget about yourself. You must practice what you preach.

Your genes affect your health and well-being; however, diet and lifestyle modification can override the genetic lottery if you're willing to make big enough changes. Those with a strong genetic predisposition to disease may have to make more dramatic changes than those with better genes. We believe nurture can trump nature.

The goal of obtaining optimum health is challenging, but it can attainable if you adhere to the basic edicts. Remember, simplicity is the marker of genius. Let's identify a simple approach to diet, exercise, sleep, and stress management in your attempt to seek optimum health.

THE ANTI-INFLAMMATORY LIFESTYLE

You must embrace an anti-inflammatory lifestyle. First, let's take a closer look at inflammation. Chronic, low-grade inflammation appears to be an underlying factor in many chronic diseases such as cardiovascular disease, diabetes, arthritis, dementia, and autoimmune diseases. The autoimmune system is effective when responding to *acute* events such as trauma and infection. However, when this defense system becomes *chronically* activated, it causes your body to identify your own tissues as a foreign invader and consequently attacks it. Damage to these tissues at a cellular level then incites additional immune responses. As a result, your immune system spins out of control in a self-perpetuating cycle of inflammation. Unfortunately, this chronic, low-grade inflammation does not alert you the way acute inflammation does with pain and erythema. The low-grade fire that propels the development of chronic disease is burning without you knowing it is there.

Chronic inflammation is initiated by "up regulation" of your genetically inherited gene pool that responds to inflammatory stimuli. The genes that tell your body to recruit an army of mediators to fight the invaders (oxidized LDL cholesterol) can run amok and lead to an over-response resulting in self-induced disease. The commonly used anti-inflammatory agents, such as non-steroidal anti-inflammatory agents (NSAIDs) and steroids, although helpful in acute settings, frequently interfere with the body's normal immune responses and may lead to serious side effects. Low-dose aspirin and statins may be beneficial; low-dose aspirin appears to lower the risk of heart attack and colon cancer through its anti-inflammatory effect.

What causes chronic inflammation? It appears that our diet and lifestyle play major roles.

Dietary Modification

Unhealthy dietary choices (high fat/high carb) play a major role in chronic inflammation, as do obesity, metabolic syndrome, smoking, hypertension, lack of exercise, chronic stress, and chronic infections. Studies show that higher intake of red and processed meats, pastries, and refined grains increases blood markers of inflammation (C- reactive protein). Alternatively, higher intake of fruit, vegetables, legumes, fish, poultry, and whole grains decrease blood markers of inflammation.

Nutrient-dense foods are composed of beneficial substances that are essential for optimal health and have the highest nutritional value. Nutrient density is defined as the amount of nutrients a food contains divided by the number of calories. When you eat high-quality foods you do not need as much to feel satisfied (satiety center in the brain is happy sooner) as opposed to the super-sized low-nutrient foods you wolf down when you rush through the fast food joint.

So let's outline the nutrient-dense foods that will allow you the greatest possibility of a victory over inflammation. The best foods for you are those high in complex carbohydrates, healthy fats, and good protein.

- **Fruits**—apples, bananas, oranges, berries, figs, kiwi, mango, and grapes
- **Vegetables**—artichokes, arugula, asparagus, broccoli, cabbage, carrots, cauliflower, celery, cucumber, eggplant, kale, sun dried tomatoes, spinach, seaweed, tomatoes, and yams
- **Grains**—high-fiber whole grain cereals, millet, oatmeal, oats, polenta, quinoa, rye, and wild rice
- **Legumes**—black beans, chickpeas, fava beans, lentils, lima beans, navy beans, pinto beans, and sprouts
- **Proteins**—egg whites, hummus, edamame, tofu, and veggie burgers

- **Foods high in Omega-3**—avocados, seeds, nuts, and fish such as wild salmon, pacific sardine, whitefish, Atlantic herring mackerel, rainbow trout, halibut, ocean perch, yellow fin tuna, blue fin tuna, and cod. (Three grams per day of most fish oils provides about 1 gram of DHA plus EPA, which is all that you require.)

Drink plenty of water to remain well-hydrated. Want something more flavorful than water and good for you? Incorporate green tea. It has many antioxidants, such as polyphenols and flavonoids, and catechins that appear to reduce risk for some chronic diseases. The polyphenols of green tea appear to have powerful antioxidant properties and scavengers for free radicals such as oxidized LDL (bad cholesterol) that damage the body's cells. Antioxidants may prevent the oxidation of LDL cholesterol. Green tea catechins have been reported to have antibacterial, anti-viral, and antifungal properties. Green tea flavonoids may improve blood sugar regulation through insulin enhancing properties. Additionally, green tea may reduce your risk for cavities. Take time for a green tea or two every day!

Also reduce sodium consumption. Salt plays a major role in high blood pressure. We have two strategies to control the concentration of sodium in our bodies:

1. Excreting the extra sodium through urine, and
2. Decreasing the intake of sodium through diet.

Young people can control sodium concentration through renal excretion because they have normal kidney function. With age, the kidneys become less efficient at excreting sodium and therefore the best option for sodium control is to reduce its consumption. The extra sodium from ingestion causes your body to retain water to maintain the proper sodium concentration in the blood serum. The increased water in your blood vessels results in increased blood pressure, which translates into increased pressure affecting the small arterioles of the kidney. This negatively affects kidney function, creating a vicious cycle where the kidneys become progressively less capable of excreting sodium. Increased sodium intake results in further increase in blood pressure promoting inflammation, and less salt ingestion results in lower blood pressure (less inflammation).

The American Medical Association recommends that healthy adults should not exceed 2,300 milligrams of sodium per day. Unfortunately, there is excessive sodium in many processed and prepackaged foods and consequently the average American is eating two to three times as much salt as is healthy.

Hypertension is in itself an epidemic disease, but it's also a risk factor for chronic inflammation which in turn promotes further disease processes. For some people with high blood pressure, decreased sodium intake is essential. If lower sodium intake is inadequate to lower blood pressure, then further steps, such as medication, will be necessary.

Exercise

Regular, moderate exercise is essential to good health and well-being. It helps maintain ideal body weight, regulates blood sugar levels, increases HDL levels (good cholesterol), and is the most underutilized anti-depressant around. Looking to your future, it may beneficially affect your genes, reverse aging at the cellular level, increase your brain power, and facilitate neurogenesis—where you grow new brain cells!

Exercise has a major effect on energy efficiency. Remember, we need energy to function well physically, mentally, and emotionally. Our cellular mitochondria are the energy source for our body's metabolism. The aging process seems to affect the efficiency of mitochondrial function at the cellular level. Studies show that regular exercise improves mitochondrial function, resulting in increased strength and functional capacity. Aerobic exercise has been shown to increase neuronal growth, and the region of the brain that grows the most is the hippocampus—the center for memory and cognition. Wow, not only will you have more energy but with regular exercise, you will think and remember better!

Regular, moderate exercise also reduces inflammation throughout your body, thus possibly affecting heart disease, cancer, autoimmune diseases, and dementia. Additionally, levels of important neurotransmitters including dopamine, serotonin, and norepinephrine are elevated in the regular exerciser. This can reduce depression, elevate mood, and enhance executive brain function.

Exercise enhances cognition for all ages. Older adults who exercise regularly remember better, handle mental tasks more efficiently, and concentrate and focus better than their sedentary friends. Young children who exercise regularly have less propensity for attention deficit disorder and learn better than those who are sedentary. Exercise also prevents obesity and all its ramifications for health and emotional well-being in the young and elderly.

Remember, the mark of genius is *simplicity*. Exercise does not have to be complicated if you choose what you like, make it fun, and do it regularly. Some people exercise best in groups and others in isolation. All types of exercises have physical and mental health benefits.

A good exercise program should incorporate aerobic, strength, and flexibility training. Aerobic exercise increases stamina and has the potential to prevent and reverse some diseases. It conditions the heart, lungs, and muscles. Aerobic exercise should be scheduled for 60 minutes a day, five days a week and should include interval training with variations in intensity. We like cycling, swimming, water walking/running, elliptical, and the step mill because they provide a maximum cardiopulmonary workout without having a negative impact on the joints over time. On the other hand, many of our friends alternate between Zumba dance, Pilates, step, and weight training classes. They find the classes to be a good workout, socially gratifying, and motivating. These classes, when rotated, offer muscle toning, core muscle strengthening, and cardiopulmonary exercises.

The rule of thumb when starting aerobic exercise is to start slow and build your aerobic capacity over time. Another caveat is to vary the program so boredom does not set in. Aerobic exercise has much value in your search for physical, emotional, and mental health.

It is critical to seek medical evaluation prior to starting an aerobic program. Your HCP can evaluate the safety of exercise from a cardiovascular perspective, including administering a stress test to identify your risk for ischemia (inadequate blood flow to the heart muscle). Determining your exercise capacity under medical supervision gives a sense of where you should begin with your aerobic exercise program.

Strength and resistance training are also critical to your overall well-being. The benefits of strength training include weight and fat loss, lower blood pressure, improved joint function/mobility, enhanced metabolism, and improved bone density. Resistance training is similar to aerobic exercise and is based on the overload principle: mildly exceed your limits to reach a new limit. The adaptation to small increases in workload (the amount of weight or number of repetitions) will allow your aerobic capacity to increase and your muscles to be stronger and have greater stamina.

Some simple tips include exercising large muscles prior to smaller muscles, doing exercises that involve multiple joints before single joints, doing difficult exercises before easy ones, and exercising the same muscle groups on alternate days. If you are new to these concepts, there is value in starting with a trainer.

Aging brings some natural loss of muscle and joint tone, but the major reason for muscle and joint stiffness is loss of flexibility. Good flexibility enhances your ability to function well in daily activities and reduces the risk for falls and injuries. The aging process results in muscle tissue, tendons, and ligaments becoming less elastic. The result is loss of flexibility. The good news is we can overcome the impact of aging with yoga, Pilates, and Zumba classes. These exercises increase upper and lower body flexibility and enhance strength and balance.

To sustain an exercise program you must choose activities you enjoy. Listen to your body—do not overdo it. Soreness, as opposed to pain, means you have pushed your muscles beyond their comfort zone (overload principle) and leads to increased strength and flexibility. You must be consistent. If you miss a day, do a little more the next day. Last but not least, exercise with family and friends to provide motivation and social support, with an added benefit of sharing time in this world of too much to do in too little time.

Additional motivation to exercise comes from research reported in the *New England Journal of Medicine* that indicates that exercise in conjunction with proper diet results in greater reductions in LDL cholesterol (the bad one that gets oxidized) than just dietary change. Also, those who exercise have less oxidation of LDL molecules than those who are sedentary. (Remember the vicious immune response started by oxidized LDL and the ultimate inflammatory response resulting in plaque formation on the artery wall.)

Stress Management

Stress negatively affects every aspect of your body and its functions. It may suppress the immune system, delay healing, increase the risk for cancer, promote inflammation, cause or exacerbate depression, lead to obesity, and affect concentration and memory. Stress also ages you faster at a cellular level. Telomeres are the DNA at the end of chromosomes that directly affect cellular aging. Cells age and die more quickly when the telomeres shorten and weaken. Interestingly, studies have shown that the levels of telomerase (the natural enzyme that repairs and restores telomeres) were lower in women with high stress levels and increased in women who followed the dietary and exercise programs we discussed earlier. Additionally, increased telomerase levels are associated with decreased LDL cholesterol in the bloodstream. This is extremely important in a world that seems to spinning out of control with stress.

One of the keys to stress management is to recognize the stress and manage it through techniques like meditation and yoga. Through such practice, you learn to control your response to the external stressors you face.

Combining exercise and meditation works well for me. The 60 minutes on the exercise step mill is a time when I meditate. I pick one focused area of thought and go off into a dream state. It makes the aerobic exercise go quickly and allows me to drift off. During this time, I often solve work or personal problems, or visualize how I want to write a conversation, as the one we are having in this book. This is my favorite time of the day. I am conditioning my body aerobically while I am recharging my mental battery and exercising my psyche muscle. This is a time when I am able to stretch my thinking beyond "road blocks." It results in a feeling of exhilaration. Elizabeth jogs outside, melting away the stresses of participating in a cardiology training program.

What can you do to manage stress? Focus on something pleasant and peaceful, quiet your mind. Practice yoga. Combine aerobic exercise and meditation. Reduce your exposure to stimulants, such as coffee and sodas. Protect your social support system—it is important to have a strong sense of connectivity and community. Reframe frustrations: things always seem different 24 hours after the fact.

Sleep

Sleep helps the body and mind recover from mental and physical fatigue. This recovery is essential to peak executive function and physical performance. Optimal executive function helps us adhere to dietary discretion and exercise rituals that lead to optimal health. Sleep is critical to our development into a health athlete.

Sleep debt affects strength, cardiovascular capacity, emotional state, cognition, and overall energy level. Reaction time, concentration, memory, and logical/analytical reasoning all decline with sleep deficit. Although our need for sleep varies depending on age, gender, and genetic profile, the consensus is that humans need a minimum of seven hours for optimal physical and mental function.

The importance of sleep is dramatically represented by the consequences of the long-standing system of training physicians. Resident physicians in training work in 36-hour shifts and often put in more than 120 hours per week. In 1984, journalist Sidney Zion brought a widely publicized lawsuit that put that system on trial after his daughter died following a visit to a New York City Hospital. A grand jury concluded that she had received suboptimal care from inexperienced interns and residents functioning on little or no sleep. (See Chapter 11 for an extensive discussion of this case.) According to the National Academy of Sciences, medical errors frequently are related to sleep deprivation and account for approximately 100,000 deaths per year.

The implications of sleep deprivation are enormous:

- Decreased Performance and Alertness: Reducing your nighttime sleep by as little as 1½ hours for just one night could result in a reduction of daytime alertness by as much as 32%.
- Memory and Cognitive Impairment: Decreased alertness and excessive daytime sleepiness impair your ability to remember, think, and process information.
- Stressed Relationships: Disruption of a bed partner's sleep due to a sleep disorder may cause significant problems for the relationship.
- Poor Quality of Life: You might be unable to participate in certain activities that require sustained attention, like going to the movies, seeing your child in a school play, or engaging in personal relationships.
- Occupational Injury: Excessive sleepiness also contributes to a more than a two-fold higher risk of sustaining an occupational injury.

- Automobile Injury: The National Highway Traffic Safety Administration estimates conservatively that each year, drowsy driving is responsible for at least 100,000 automobile crashes, 71,000 injuries, and 1,550 fatalities.
- Decreased Work Potential: Lack of ability to sustain concentration can affect one's ability to be productive.

Play

Our memories of our youth are filled with images of play, whether it was playing peekaboo with a parent, making a cardboard box into a spaceship, or playing hide and seek with friends. Unfortunately as we evolved into adulthood, we were told that we were too old to play and have fun. Work was the priority. Yet it's during play that our imagination can spark true creativity. Interestingly, it was during a break from work that Watson and Crick stumbled upon the double-helix shape that comprises the fundamental structure of DNA!

Play is essential. It allows us to do something for pure joy and not as a means to an end. Play is important for our health, for our emotional recovery, and for building essential loving relationships. Play is an antidote to stress, and stress, as we all know, is the enemy of creativity, curiosity, and productivity. Take time to play every day so you can let your inner child feel the positive emotions that drive the key breakthroughs in thinking. Play is not only a childhood activity, it is essential to *every adult, every day.*

— ELIZABETH'S THOUGHTS —

The components of a balanced life—eating healthy, exercising, resting, and playing—are concepts that we probably consider *common sense.* Yet, we don't practice them. I, myself, am guilty of not practicing all of these elements and that's because of lack of recognition, discipline, and time management.

Recognition is the process of taking a subset of information that we hear or read about in our life from the periphery, bringing it to the forefront of our minds, and making a firm decision to bring it to fruition. It's taking what you read in this chapter and actively deciding for yourself that "this is what I'm going to do" rather than passively reading the information and thinking "I should probably do this." Instead of just acknowledging that you should eat healthy and exercise, take the time to make a meal plan or schedule workouts into your daily activities.

Discipline is necessary to carry out these plans you've invested time in making. It is hard to not reach for "comfort foods" such as cookies, chips, ice cream, or fast foods when you're hungry and on a time crunch. I am very much guilty of this and in fact have quite a sweet tooth. (Tim can attest to this "weakness" as he occasionally has to help with my personal "discipline" by taking away the sweet treat!) It's equally hard to exercise when you're exhausted from work. This is where discipline comes in. It's the ability to make a choice at lunch time that you're going to have a salad rather fried chicken or a hamburger. It's the ability to push yourself to work out rather than collapse on the couch and watch television.

Time management skills help you achieve your goals for a healthy life. One of the adages I try to practice is *"Don't just work harder, work smarter."* This means working efficiently to complete necessary tasks so you can get home at a reasonable time and allow yourself time for exercise, rest, and play. Essentialism is defining your tasks or goals at work so you can accomplish the things you need to do for your personal well-being.

Effective time management at home can allow you to prepare yourself mentally and physically to be efficient at work. For example, instead of exercising on your own, ask a friend, significant other, or family member to join you. That way, workouts not only become more enjoyable, they allow you to spend time with an important person in your life. If you prefer to work out on your own, pick an activity such as running or yoga that can allow you to free your mind and decompress.

When they start medical school, most people are in their 20s and many are just out of college, where they lived on fast food, pizzas, Ramen noodles, and frozen dinners. That kind of diet, along with a sedentary lifestyle, will suddenly catch up to them as their metabolism becomes sluggish with age. I have seen many people who were skinny during college quickly gain weight by the end of medical school or during training. Stress causes the body to release steroid hormones that further promote weight gain. You must take the time to slow down and plan a more deliberate, healthy life and prevent yourself from eventually spiraling down a road of obesity and disease.

CHAPTER 4

Family—Living a Life that Really Matters

"In the end, you'll know which people really love you. They're the ones who see you for who you are and no matter what, always find a way to be at your side."

Randy K. Milholland

— TIM'S THOUGHTS —

The essential life requires that you embrace your family as your number one priority, followed by your own personal health and then your work. When I need a reminder of this hierarchy, I think of a close friend of my mine whose son died at age 18. He realized he never took the time to know his own son because he was too busy with his career. He had been too busy to do homework with his son and to watch his sports games. He missed teacher conferences and evening meals. My close friend was left empty.

At the very end, everything else will pale in comparison to the love of your family—your parents, grandparents, siblings, and the family you build with your partner. They are the most important essentials in your life.

The essentials of your family will be challenged by your work and by those you work for during the course of your career. You will be told that in order for you to meet the demands and expectations of your occupation and your bosses, your family must be secondary to work. Never succumb to such illogical thinking. We both have endured criticism for putting our family first. A family first mentality does not equate to a failed career. I knew my sons and they knew me.

Can you put family first and still succeed in the work force? Absolutely. The key is essentialism. Identify exactly what you want for yourself and your family. Learn to say *no*. Have you ever felt a tension between what you wanted to do and what you were being pressured to do? Have you ever said *yes* when you really wanted to say *no* because you wanted to avoid friction, conflict, or demotion? Have you ever been afraid to turn down the request of a boss, professor, friend, or colleague? The ability to say *no*, especially when *no* is the correct response, can be challenging. *No* means we could miss an opportunity, stir things up, or burn bridges. But failing to say *no* may have far deeper consequences.

A high school friend, Jenny, told me that when she was 12 years old, she and her father made grand plans for a ski trip to Breckenridge in conjunction with one of her father's lectures. They would ski, go shopping and sightseeing, and eat dinner by the fireplace in the lodge. Jenny eagerly anticipated this weekend with her father for months. That day finally arrived. Father and daughter traveled to Breckenridge and Jenny attended her father's lecture, waiting anxiously at the back of the room so they could escape to the slopes before her father was barraged with questions. As they were leaving the convention center, her dad was beckoned by a college friend and business associate who invited Jenny and her father to dinner that night. As Jenny's father responded that "dinner sounded great," Jenny's heart crumbled into pieces. Then her father continued, "But not tonight, because Jenny and I have a date." Jenny's dad grabbed her hand and they spent a memorable day and evening of father-daughter fun. Jenny knew that she was first on her father's list of priorities.

You may be approached by people who want you to perform duties to their advantage in exchange for possible promotions or favors. Evaluate these situations carefully and remember the importance of a simple *no* if it will interfere with one of your essential priorities. Even if things in your career do not go in the direction you had anticipated or hoped, other opportunities may be awaiting you. In his book: *Zero to One*, Peter Thiel tells a great personal story about being on a traditional path that was carved out for him. He attended Stanford for undergraduate school and then matriculated to Stanford law school. He clerked on a federal appeals court for one year and was invited to interview for clerkships with Supreme Court Justices Kennedy and Scalia. When he did not get the clerkships, he was devastated. Rather than dwelling on his losses, he went on to become an entrepreneur and venture capitalist who developed and sold PayPal.

Remember, there is no one path. Talented people survive and do well, no matter what adversarial event is thrown at them. You don't have to compromise your values or sell your soul to the devil to advance in your career. Make your priorities and stick with them. Don't let others use you for their own benefit. Trust in yourself and invest in yourself and your family. The rest will work itself out.

— ELIZABETH'S THOUGHTS —

When you're young, you think you know everything. As you get older, you really start to appreciate the wisdom of your parents and the importance of family. Over the years, I've been blessed to enrich my life with many good people I've come to call friends. However, with major life changes—marriages, children, jobs, or moving—we would spend less time together. It is part of the natural processes of living. Though my friends and I gather together on occasions when time permits, we all have a mutual understanding of the importance of family.

The medical career path is a tough one with its own set of unique challenges at each stage. During each rough patch, I constantly found myself reaching out to my family. They've been an incredible foundation that I came to appreciate even more through the rigors of medical training. I am forever grateful for my family for being supportive through the tough times and keeping me grounded. It is through their understanding and support that I have made it as far as I have.

CHAPTER 5

Take Time for Introspection

— ELIZABETH'S THOUGHTS —

Life can become very complicated, very quickly. To prevent yourself from losing perspective, take time for introspective reflection to figure out your own needs and wants, and how they will affect your present and future pursuits. This is a necessity at every stage of the process to becoming a well adjusted, happy physician.

During your formative years in high school or college, before you even embark on the path to becoming a physician, you must ask yourself if you have the mental fortitude and desire for the field to take on an arduous journey of schooling and training. Once in medical school, you must evaluate which medical specialty would be compatible with your personality, wants, and needs. During residency, you need to decide if you want to pursue a subspecialty fellowship, or if you want to be done with training and just go to practice. You also need to determine the type of job setting in which you want to work: academic or private, inpatient or outpatient.

The path to becoming a physician is not a well-paved interstate with a clear, smooth drive. Rather, it's more of a gravel road on a hiker's path up a mountain with twists and turns that you need to carefully consider before you take them, lest you get lost. However, like a nature hike, it can be a pleasant experience if it's well thought out and you are prepared.

First and foremost, be *realistic*. Think about your personal strengths and weaknesses. Decide what you can and absolutely cannot change. What are your capabilities and can you improve on them? A person whose parents are both doctors may have early exposure to clinical knowledge, but if that person is unmotivated, he or she may not succeed. A person from an impoverished background who has ambition and dedication may excel exponentially in the field.

Don't work on idealistic plans only to be disappointed when they do not come to fruition. For example, let's look at the process to get into medical school. The ideal, well-rounded candidates that all medical schools seek are those who demonstrate academic excellence, a charismatic personality, and active involvement in community service. However, with the sheer number of applications medical schools receive during interview season, it is not possible for interview board members to look in detail at the qualifications of all its applicants. Instead, they have a cut-off for grade point average (GPA) and medical college admission test (MCAT) scores. Applicants who have GPAs and MCAT scores above the cut-off criteria will be more seriously considered for an interview; those below the cut-off point likely will receive a letter declining them for an interview. So if you're applying to medical school, but your GPA or MCAT is subpar, you may need to take some time to assess whether you can improve on these two aspects and how you're going to do it.

Once you get into medical school, you'll notice a recurring theme of objective cut-offs. Along the way, you will need to take additional board tests, and your scores on these boards will define your chosen medical specialty path. Certain subspecialties such as dermatology or plastic surgery are much more competitive and will require outstanding résumés, pristine medical school GPAs, exceptional board scores, and countless extracurricular and academic activities.

While reflecting, keep in mind the element of trade-offs as discussed in Chapter 1. Some professions require more time commitment than others. If you have a family with whom you'd like to spend more time, a specialty such as general surgery with its arduous training hours and calls may prevent you from doing that.

Your option is to pick another less-demanding profession or, if it's something you truly want, sacrifice some time with your family. It's not impossible to complete a taxing residency and take care of your obligations to your family, and many have successfully traveled down this difficult road.

However, each of us is different with our own sets of strengths, weaknesses, and goals. Define what yours are and set realistic expectations for yourself and your family.

Also, keep in mind that the journey through the medical field is a dynamic one. During the course of my residency training, there was a cardiothoracic surgery resident who had an accomplished medical career as an anesthesiologist, yet there he was, doing a surgical residency. During medical school, he had aspirations to become a surgeon. However, when his wife became pregnant, he realized he did not want to be in a specialty where he would not have time to be home with his family. He decided to do anesthesiology and went on to practice that for many years. During his years of practice as an anesthesiologist, he yearned to be on the other side of the sterile curtain doing the surgeries himself. When his children were grown, despite having an established life as an anesthesia attending, he made the ultimate decision to go back to residency training for general surgery. He went on to do a fellowship in cardiothoracic training. His story demonstrates the level of assessment and re-assessment necessary not only during the training years, but during practice to accommodate the changes life sends our way.

Take time for personal reflection to not only make decisions pertaining to your career, but to also cultivate your character. Oftentimes, during the hustle and bustle of busy schooling, training, or working hours, it is easy to lose sight of what the practice of medicine really means. This will only be exacerbated by the expectations of the present-day medical bureaucracy that emphasizes quantity rather than true quality for compensation.

A friend of mine during residency candidly shared with me the incident that made him realize his disillusionment with medicine and disappointment with himself as a person. During his internship year, after a long stretch of hard months and endless hours at the hospital, he gradually disconnected himself from his patients. His eagerness to help patients and learn all that he could about them and their ailments slowly dissipated and in its place came resentment.

He continued on this way until an especially difficult call night on the medical intensive care unit (MICU). He was going on his 18th hour of work without sleep and admitting the 12th sick patient who was going to need a central line and on the verge of requiring intubation. While setting up for these procedures, he was getting a barrage of pages from various nurses on the unit about the other MICU patients. Battling exhaustion, he returned the pages and continued on with the procedures—all the while wondering, "When will this all end?" Then he received another page. It was the nurse taking care of one of the patients he had admitted earlier. The patient had died. Rather than feeling sad, he felt a sense of *relief* and mild joy. One less patient he would have to deal with for the night—*thank goodness.*

After 28 hours of work, he went home and collapsed. After some sleep, he reflected on the previous night call and felt incredible guilt for the sense of relief he felt at the exchange rate of a life. This realization opened his eyes. He made it through the rest of his internship year the best he could, but after many other moments of self-reflection realized his character was slowly being overwhelmed by the demands and stress of work. He ultimately decided to leave internal medicine and has felt much more at peace with himself.

When entering into medicine, we focus on the glorified aspects of being a physician—the altruistic doctor saving lives and living the dream—glamorized by society and the media. The reality, especially with the trend toward commercialized medicine, is that the medical field can quickly become a self-promoting profession coursing toward a robotic decision-making processes in order to meet reimbursement quotas or to avoid litigation. With expectations that physicians take on higher patient loads yet still allot the "proper" amount of time with the patient, combined with the constant bombardment of documentation, it is no wonder that many physicians report burnout.

You may find yourself immersed in the vast sea of the medical field and it becomes very easy to adopt a "sink, swim, or die" attitude of survival. However, this is not the road to maintain character, let alone develop it.

Part Two

The Journey to Becoming a Healthcare Provider

CHAPTER 6

The Medical Educational Process

— TIM'S EXPERIENCE —

During this period of intense education, each person is developing the intellectual, emotional, and social intelligence to become a healthcare detective/sleuth, deep thinker, and problem solver. The following discussion is based in large part on my experiences in medical school. I hope it helps prepare you for success.

ACCEPTANCE TO MEDICAL SCHOOL

Acceptance to medical school elicits intense emotions of pure joy and immense pride, accomplishment, and security. The future appears bright for those who are about to embark on a professional career filled with opportunity and financial security When medical school classes begin, the initial sense of pride and confidence is often replaced by anxiety and uncertainty. The impending fear of failure overwhelms the hijacked amygdala as the start of classes approaches.

What if I am not smart enough to compete against my "brainiac" classmates?

What was I thinking when I decided to go to medical school given the sacrifices I must make?

Will I have any time for family, friends, and leisure?

Maybe my friends who were rejected are the real winners.

These fears are real, intimidating, and must be overcome to be successful in medical school.

First, be assured that the medical school would not have accepted you had they not believed you would be successful. It's rare that accepted individuals do not pass the curriculum—the exception typically involving unique circumstances that prevent the student from remaining in medical school.

Second, let me reassure you that you can cope with the amount of information you must absorb in medical school under the given time constraints and still have family and friend time, and time for leisure activities. How? You do it by adopting being essential—applying a well-defined, systematic approach to each aspect of your life, as discussed in Chapter 1.

PRIORITIZING ESSENTIALS

Let's take a journey that elucidates a strategic approach to success with medical school, family and friends, and leisure time.

When you said *yes* to your acceptance letter, you elected medical school as an essential in your life for the next four years. The study of medicine became a priority. The decision to say *yes* has implications for the other components of your life as well. The Latin root of the word *decision* means "to cut." You need to reduce or even eliminate activities, relationships, and life options that you truly enjoy, but that would interfere with the time and energy needed to master the complex subjects encountered in medical school. If that commitment seems onerous, you have made the wrong decision. There are trade-offs that cannot be denied, even by the most keen minds.

Prioritizing essentials is mandatory once you enter the medical field. Personally, I believe your family should be your utmost priority. The beauty of family is they will be most accepting and understanding of your essentialist soul that says you must miss a family gathering or social engagement because of school work. Family will always provide emotional and financial support and understanding when you face overwhelming time and energy constraints. They will provide unconditional love when you need it most.

Prioritizing friendships is a different matter and may require deep thought. Social relationships are critical to our individual sense of emotional harmony and to our happiness. True friends are analogous to family and therefore of utmost importance. They will understand your time and energy constraints and will accept your decision to defer social engagements.

The key here is the difference between friends and true friends. The latter is difficult to define and varies at different stages of life, but you must develop the skill and astuteness to identify and separate true friends from friends. This is challenging because at the age of average medical students, relationships are often immature and filled with jealousy, spite, and irrational actions. The process of eliminating friends takes courage. We worry that the loss of a friend may result in us missing out on a great opportunity. We are fearful of "stirring the pot," burning bridges, or tarnishing our reputation and being perceived as thinking we are better than someone else. We don't want to hurt someone we like.

But deciding you lack the time to maintain a relationship does not make you a bad person. Steve Jobs said it well: "*Deciding what not to do is as important as deciding what to do.*" Saying *yes* and then failing to meet commitments leads to anger, frustration, and often emotionally painful break ups. In addition, failing to say *no* to relationships that are not essential may deter you from achieving other essential goals. Letting go of relationships requires careful soul searching, deep thought, and upfront discussions as to why you will not be able to meet the demands of the relationship.

The new boundaries are empowering and protect your time from being hijacked by someone else's agenda. The elimination of high-maintenance people who tend to make their problems your problems is essential because it prevents you from being distracted from your purposes. Simply and succinctly stated, you must eliminate whoever is siphoning off your time and energy for their own purpose. When we don't set up clearly identified, demarcated boundaries in our lives, we can end up imprisoned by the intrusions of others. The boundaries are sources of liberation to explore our chosen areas of interest.

Go with your gut instinct. The friends you maintain must understand and respect the carefully crafted social contract you discuss—the boundaries of the relationship. There must be an upfront discussion of the time and energy constraints that may affect your friendship. The idea of enforcing limits becomes easier and effortless with time and practice.

Protecting one's assets is also essential. We are the greatest asset we can contribute to family, friends, and society. If we underinvest in our minds, bodies, and emotional well-being, we minimize the tools we need to make our highest contribution to the people most important to us.

THE DIDACTIC YEARS—YEARS 1 AND 2

The first year of medical school is both scary and exciting. The fear of not succeeding that is prevalent at the beginning of the year fades as students become immersed in a broad range of interesting topics, such as biochemistry, cell biology, embryology, genetics, immunology, physiology, and neuroscience. Then there are the interdisciplinary courses in physiology and neuroscience, as well as courses in cell biology, human behavior, and psychopathology. There is a constant infusion through the first year of clinical ethics in medicine and an introduction to critical thinking. This overall blend of courses allows students to begin assessing molecular and cellular body function. The concept of structure and function is well developed.

The course work during the didactic years is challenging, but the insights gained are lifelong learning tools.

Year 1 Courses

Human Anatomy. The human anatomy course presents the gross structure and function of the human body as it relates to the practice of medicine. By using surface and cadaver anatomy, students acquire a three-dimensional understanding of structural relationships in the living body. Working in groups, students dissect the major structures of the body. Prosections and demonstration specimens provide amplification and clarification. Laboratory sessions are supplemented by sessions in which radiological techniques are used to illustrate parts of the bony structures and the abdominopelvic viscera. There is a correlation between the anatomical study and its relationship to medical practice.

Medical Biochemistry. The medical biochemistry course introduces students to the fundamentals of modern molecular biology and biochemistry as it applies to the practice of medicine. The first block of learning in biochemistry helps students understand proteins at the molecular level and their relationship to structure and function. Typically, there is an exploration of the basic amino acid building blocks and how differences in structural architecture are manifest in different functional states and disease states. Then there is an exploration of nucleic acids, macromolecular machinery, and the regulatory factors at the molecular level. Study of the intrinsic nature of metabolism includes the fundamentals of carbohydrate and amino acid metabolism, including some interesting disease states arising from disruption of the metabolic machinery, including the role of genetics and environment.

Finally, there is an exhaustive exploration of lipid metabolism and its relationship to disease states that are commonly identified in clinical medicine. The introduction to lipid metabolism allows an exploration of common disease states, including diabetes and the metabolic syndrome, obesity, and the number one cause of death in men and women: coronary artery disease.

Histology. Histology—the study of cell and tissue biology—is covered in lectures and coordinated laboratory sessions that introduce the detailed structure and function of cells, tissues, and organ systems of the human body. These features of cells and tissues are highlighted with the use of light and electron microscopy. There is a strong emphasis on the structural and functional relationships between different cell types in human cells and tissues with an emphasis on how alterations in cellular architecture and cellular behavior can result in various disease states.

Initially, students learn the functional morphology of cells and their organelles, the biochemical composition of cellular components and products, the unique features of cell surfaces and cellular movement, and the basics of cell-cell and cell-matrix interactions. Then there is a systematic survey of the body's organ systems emphasizing the specialized cell types in each organ system.

Embryology. Embryology studies embryologic development from ovulation to birth with an emphasis on the embryology of the major organ systems. There is an integration of the embryologic topics with human anatomy to facilitate the understanding of anatomical relationships, selected birth defects, and genotype to phenotype heterogeneity resulting in anatomic variants. CD-ROM animation of embryologic development allows a critical visualization of embryologic changes in real time. The key focus is on embryology's relevance to developmental biology and medicine.

Genomics. The future of medicine is genomics and first-year medical students begin with genetics. There is an introduction to basic principles of human genetics and its application to clinical medicine. The introduction to chromosome abnormalities, genetic patterns of inheritance, inborn errors of metabolism, multifactorial inheritance, population genetics, gene mapping and identification, genetic screening, gene therapy, and ethical issues surrounding genetic selection makes this course feel very clinical and exciting. It is the future of medicine and the foundation for prevention.

Immunology. First-year students learn the components of the immune system, their locations in the human body, and their action and reaction in health and disease, as well as how the immune system identifies and attempts to eliminate pathogens, how certain pathogens elude the immune system and cause disease, and how the immune system can mistake normal cells as foreign and initiate disease.

The course is fascinating because students are introduced to the genes and molecules that play essential roles in the immune system as it defends the body. The central players include antigens, antigen receptors, antibodies, complement, major histocompatibility complex loci, chemokine, and cytokines. Students explore the interactions that result in innate disease and acquired disease. Ultimately, they explore immune deregulation. Interventions including vaccines, immunomodulators, hypersensitivities, immunodeficiency, autoimmunity, graft versus host disease, transplant immunology, and tumor immunology. The level of clinical significance makes the course stimulating and relevant to future studies across a wide range of disciplines.

Human behavior. Human behavior is interesting because it introduces students to the basic science of human psychology that is relevant to understanding aberrant behaviors and mental disorders. The exploration of human psychosocial development and the underpinnings of human behavior in relationship to disease and health are reviewed. There is an in-depth exploration of human response to disease states from the perspective of the patient, the family, and the physician.

Physiology. Physiology examines physiologic function of major organ systems of the body. Topics include membranes; transport systems; skeletal, smooth, and cardiac muscle; and the physiologic function of the cardiovascular, respiratory, renal, gastrointestinal, and endocrine systems. There is an in-depth exploration of the physiologic function of all major organ systems of the human body.

Neuroscience. Neuroscience reinforces all the concepts encountered thus far. Students study the principles of cellular physiology and cellular excitability to specialized cells of the nervous system and their synaptic connections. The study of neuroanatomical features of the nervous system and relevant clinical correlations makes the course pertinent to clinical medicine. Then the course explores sensory, motor, and cognitive systems, and introduces the neurological examination, which requires an in-depth understanding of neuroanatomy and neurophysiology,

Year 2 Courses

Year two is as exciting, or more so, than year one. The second year curriculum integrates the disciplines of clinical medicine, pathology, microbiology, and pharmacology. The course work introduces second year students to the general principles of cardiology, pulmonary, renal, hematopoietic, musculoskeletal, gastrointestinal, and central and peripheral nervous systems, and extremes of life. Each discipline reviews the pharmcokinetics, genetics, and neoplastic components of the system. This systems approach to teaching and learning allows a broad integration of the major topics that will be pertinent in the clerkship years.

Clinical Medicine. Clinical medicine offers principles in a classroom setting that serve as a transition from basic to clinical medicine. The goal is to introduce students to the skills necessary to participate in clinical medicine. Didactic teaching materials reinforce the pathophysiology of human diseases, the differential diagnosis of cardinal symptoms of the different organ systems, and how to approach them clinically. Students learn how to gather clinical data, how to evaluate the data with expert clinical reasoning and judgment, as well as how to interpret the data in light of the patient's clinical status. There is a strong emphasis on ethical behavior and professionalism, the idea being that it is an honor to care for the well-being of patients.

Pharmacology. Pharmacology is approached initially as a basic biomedical science, but in the second year the focus turns to clinical pharmacology and clinical therapeutics. Students develop a strong understanding of pharmacodynamics and pharmacokinetics, and the pharmacologic and toxicological properties of the major classes of drugs. There is a strong emphasis on understanding the mechanisms of drug-induced modifications of physiologic function of the various organ systems, and consideration is given to drug interactions and dosing based on the function of all the human organ systems.

Medical Microbiology. Medical microbiology introduces students to the importance of microorganisms in disease processes, and infectious disease syndromes caused by the various microorganisms. Students learn the biology of viruses, bacteria, fungi, and eukaryotic organisms, and their mechanisms of pathogenesis. Then, there is a focus on organ-specific pathology caused by infectious agents. The fundamental concepts are building blocks to the principles that are used by infectious disease specialists.

Anatomic and Clinical Pathology. Anatomic and clinical pathology provide the etiology, pathogenesis, and pathophysiology of general disease processes and specific diseases of organ systems. The opportunity to participate in autopsy reviews allows a synthesis of the clinical condition, anatomy, imaging, and pathology. This is a unique opportunity to view the entire spectrum of a disease process and reassess whether there were any issues not considered when caring for the patient. The process reinforces the continual learning curve that physicians face in clinical medicine and reinforces the limitations of our diagnostic capacity and therapeutic options.

ACLS. Advanced cardiac life support (ACLS) is a second-year course that includes didactic information about the management of cardiac arrest, including rhythm recognition, drug use, cardiac defibrillators, and the latest protocols used to perform ACLS. The course has practice skills for airway management, assessment and treatment of various dysrhythmias including bradycardia, tachycardia, ventricular tachycardia/fibrillation, asystole, and pulseless electrical activity.

Reflecting on the early years makes me smile. It was a fun and fascinating time. The course work was interesting and established the ground work that I use to this very day. The professors in the basic science years are scholars dedicated to their discipline. They are fully committed to teaching and helping students absorb the vast array of information. Although at times the amount of work seems daunting, different courses piece together like a puzzle and result in a big picture that allows you to be prepared for clinical rotations.

Helping each other survive the marathon of learning solidifies the friendships you develop during these "trying times." The team approach to learning is the foundation for how you will practice medicine in later life. Friendships built in the "survival mode" seem to be long-lasting.

THE CLERKSHIP YEARS—YEARS 3 AND 4

The third and fourth years are exciting because they involve direct patient care.

Year 3 Rotations

The third year typically includes rotations through family medicine, internal medicine, neurology, obstetrics and gynecology, pediatrics, psychiatry, and surgery. Throughout these rotations, students are exposed to inpatient and outpatient clinical experiences. It is exhilarating, as you feel like a **"real" doctor**.

Family Medicine: The family medicine clerkship exposes students to primary care role models and ambulatory clinical experiences in healthcare delivery away from the tertiary care setting. Students work with family medicine physicians who are excited to share their experience and knowledge. The patients come from a broad demographic and allow students to observe and learn about gender, culture, and race in relationship to health and disease.

Internal Medicine: Internal medicine involves hospital-based experiences and rotation through the ambulatory care center. Under the supervision of a house staff resident and an attending physician, students are responsible for admission workups, progress reports, oral presentations, and the ongoing care of assigned patients.

The objective of the internal medicine clerkship is to develop proficiency in how to approach the diagnosis after a comprehensive history and physical examination and to begin to understand how to make therapeutic decisions for serious medical illnesses, to foster an appreciation and understanding of disease as an expression of deranged physiology, and to inculcate habits of critical inquiry and self-education.

Students begin to understand the physician's responsibility to the patient—the responsibility to act as a fiduciary for the patient. Teaching is carried out with house staff and attending physicians on hospital rounds and at lectures and conferences specifically aimed at the clerks. The students' job is to be curious and to be prepared to answer the questions that surface.

Neurology: A comprehensive and intense neurology rotation offers instruction and understanding across a wide spectrum of complex neurological diseases, with emphasis on diagnosis and management. The rotation is cognitively challenging. The spectrum of neurological diseases is challenging, as the diagnosis can be subtle and the therapeutic options often limited. The integration and synthesis of the medical history and the neurological physical examination can be challenging and often is a brain teaser for the non-expert in neurological disease.

Obstetrics and Gynecology: Obstetrics and gynecology is a rotation split between the two. During obstetrics, students rotate though postpartum and antepartum care and learn about the medical complications of pregnancy. The really exciting experience is delivering babies of uncomplicated pregnancies under the guidance of the resident and supervising staff. During gynecology rotation, students work in a gynecology clinic and participate in surgeries. They receive didactic lectures from the house staff and the attending physician.

Pediatrics: Pediatrics is in the inpatient and outpatient setting. Students are members of a clinical management team under the supervision of a pediatric resident and full-time attending that allows for clinical learning through patient care and didactic teaching. They are expected to take initial histories, perform initial physical examinations, and prepare progress notes. Students present their clinical history, physical examination findings, and clinical impression of the patient as well as a plan of evaluation and care to the resident and attending physician. This allows immediate feedback and on-the-spot learning.

The rotation in pediatrics is designed to emphasize normal growth and development and the impact of disease on the child and the family.

Additionally, there is a major emphasis on the prevention of disease and injury and the importance of establishing healthy living habits early in life.

Psychiatry: Psychiatry is an important rotation that introduces the evolving doctors to complex mental illness that they may confront in inpatient psychiatry, consultation/liaison psychiatry, and community health and well-being. The experience is eye-opening as students begin to understand the complex nature of mental illness, ranging from depression to schizophrenia. There is a strong emphasis on the diagnosis of mental disorders and the biopsychosocial treatment of the various psychiatric disorders.

Surgery: The third-year surgical clerkship is designed to introduce students to the theoretical and practical aspects of surgical patient care. Emphasis is placed on the underlying pathophysiology rather than the technical aspects of surgical procedures. Students are actively involved in the daily care of surgical patients and diagnostic and therapeutic decision making. The rotation is an introduction to a complex field that either grabs the students as their future career or brings them to the realization that they are not cut out for the world of surgery.

Year 4 Rotations

During the fourth year, students complete rotations that prepare them for internship by selecting from a variety of specialties in acute care, ambulatory care, and sub-internships through the subspecialties. The elective options allow them to explore their interests and provide an opportunity to visit other medical institutions in different parts of the country—ideally programs where they would like to intern. Applications for internship/residency typically are completed early in the fourth year of medical school.

Personality often influences whether students want acute care type settings or ambulatory care settings for their future career. It is important to find out where you feel comfortable and happy. The various rotations will often cement the preconceived notions or sway the evolving doctor in a different direction. You must feel comfortable in your own skin when in a practice setting.

Acute Care: The acute care rotation offers instruction in the diagnosis and management of acutely ill or injured patients. This type of exposure is found in the intensive care unit, critical care unit, and the emergency room.

During this rotation, fourth-year medical students function as integral members of a medical or surgical team, providing a high level of care to acutely ill or injured patients. Under the medical supervision of residents, fellows, and attending physicians, the medical students gain an enhanced knowledge of stabilizing, resuscitating, and managing acutely ill patients. This exposure is exciting for some students and anxiety-provoking for others.

Ambulatory Care: Ambulatory care is an out-patient clinic experience where patients are evaluated for less-acute illnesses. A strong emphasis is place on promoting health and prevention. The opportunity to learn how to motivate patients toward healthy living through exercise and diet is crucial. The epidemics of obesity, metabolic syndrome, and coronary artery disease could all be reversed through education and coaching in the ambulatory setting.

Medicine Sub-Internship: Medicine sub-internship is a unique opportunity to explore your interests. This can be done in pediatrics, surgery, internal medicine, and obstetrics and gynecology, to name a few. It is an important time to identify where you feel at home. It is imperative that you find your niche and don't try to satisfy someone else's dream, whether that is mentor, parents, or family. You're the one who must go to work every day.

ON REFLECTION

Reflecting on my clerkship years makes me realize how lucky I was during that fun and fascinating time. I loved the various rotations and found all clerkships stimulating and an excellent learning experience. I was fortunate to have great teachers who motivated me to absorb new information every day. I found routines that made me feel well emotionally, physically, and mentally.

Russell Wilson of the Seattle Seahawks says: "the separation between winning and not winning is the level of preparation." I could not agree more. Whatever rotation I was on, I prepared like it would be my future. I believe every chief resident believed I would join their specialty. I immersed myself in the rotation to get the greatest return on my investment of time and energy.

Every evening, I prepared for the next day. I ate dinner then studied for two hours. Next, I hit the pavement for a 10-mile run—often in frigid conditions. During the run, I reviewed in my mind all the things I had studied the previous two hours. At the end of my run, I took a hot shower to relax, then wrote down all the material I had covered and compared it to my notes. This allowed me to reinforce the information so I could present the material on rounds without cue cards.

This was my regimen seven days a week. It worked well for me physically, emotionally, and mentally. I believe the key to mastery of large amounts of complex concepts is a regimented routine—a throwback from my training as a college basketball player. This is not the only approach, but an approach that worked well for me. No matter what approach you pursue, you must eat well, exercise, and get adequate rest.

My future was identified when I did a rotation at the Mayo Clinic in Rochester, Minnesota. I went there without a true purpose—I simply wanted to see the institution and experience the medical environment at what was always identified in my youth as the greatest medical care institution in the world.

I arrived and met the residents running the service. They included me from day one as though I were family. The variety of patients and the teaching by the residents, fellows, and staff was beyond my wildest dreams. The staff critically reviewed my history and physical examination skills and gave me immediate feedback and instruction. When my housing didn't work out, one of the residents invited me to live at his house for the month.

The four weeks went by like a flash. I knew I needed to train in Rochester. I returned home and prayed nightly that I would be accepted into the internal medicine program at Mayo–Rochester. I was accepted and it laid the foundation of my medical career.

— ELIZABETH'S EXPERIENCE —

With advances in biomedical technology, pharmacology, and surgical interventions, the medical field is an ever-evolving profession and, accordingly, medical education and training are ever-evolving as well. For example, in the medical school curriculum there is a shift from traditional subject-based learning toward a more integrative or systems-based learning.

Dr. Paterick details his medical school experience from a traditional medical school curriculum in which subjects, starting with subjects taught didactically. This approach allows each student to acquire the basic Foundation of knowledge in normal anatomy, physiology, histology, and biochemistry. Pathophysiology is layered on next with pharmacology, and basic science knowledge is then applied during the clinical or clerkship years through interactions with real patients in the hospital or outpatient setting.

During my time in medical school, the traditional subject-based curriculum was still the dominant blueprint of medical education for the majority of medical schools across the nation. The blocks of topics and order in which they progressed during my first and second year of medical school were uncannily similar to those described by Dr. Paterick, with only a few deviations.

With the proliferation of medical research and clinical trials, greater emphasis was placed on medical decision-making processes that are supported by more empirical research data. From this stemmed evidence-based medicine (EBM), which promotes clinical practice and decision-making substantiated by available research data. In this course, medical students are taught the basics of medically relevant research terminology and statistical analysis.

The types of epidemiologic studies from randomized control trials (RCTs), meta-analyses, case-control, or cohort studies and strength of evidence that can be derived from each type of study are delineated in EBM. With the exorbitant amount of research data available, review and intellectual digestion of publications and statistical information can quickly become overwhelming. The EBM courses teach medical students how to search strategically for articles that are clinically relevant or applicable to their patient problem or clinical questions. Basic methods of statistical analysis as well as measures of medical statistics—sensitivity, specificity, positive/negative predictive values, and likelihood ratios—are discussed during this course as well.

During my time in medical school, interspersed between classes of the didactic first and second year, were multiple sessions involving principles of clinical medicine. It was a chance for us to play "pretend doctor." During these sessions, we were taught the clinical skills involved in taking the medical history as well as doing the physical examination. Hired actors played patients and we asked the questions necessary to elicit a good history pertaining to their presenting problem or complaint and then practiced our physical exam skills. This course provided early exposure to the complexities of the patient-physician interaction in a more controlled environment. Our simulated patients not only had a variety of medical ailments, they also displayed a variety of emotions, ranging from happy and anxious to sad and even furious. These sessions provided invaluable experiences that would help us during the third and fourth years of clerkship when we interacted with actual patients in the healthcare setting.

The new integrated or systems-based curriculum expands the boundaries of traditional disciplines or topics into contextual or issued-based applications that allow students to make connections across the disciplines. Topics are based on systems—neurology, pulmonary, cardiovascular, musculoskeletal, etc.—rather than the traditional topics of anatomy, history, physiology, etc. An example of an integrated curriculum is provided in Figure 1.

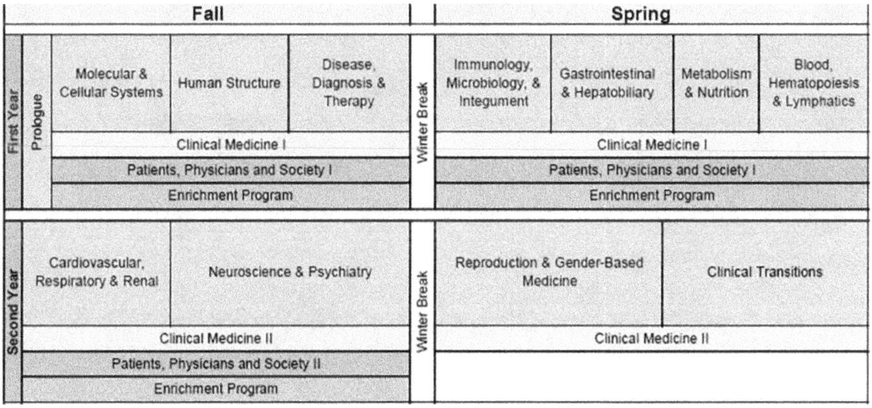

Figure 1.

Though I have not personally experienced this curriculum, one of the notable advantages is the ability to connect information with application. When an abundance of knowledge is thrusted on medical students in the first and second year of medical school, a common question is, "why do I have to learn this?" While listening to a lecture on the entire biochemical cascade of the complement system and chemokines involved in the different types of pathways of immune response, students might be inclined to ask, "Why should I care about this?"

An integrated approach to the curriculum answers that question. After they learn the normal immune response, students can extend this knowledge to clinical pathologies of immune hyperactivity (autoimmune disorders, cancers), immune-deficiencies (HIV/AIDS, complement deficiency), and therapeutics (immunosuppressants for transplant and rheumatologic disorders). Part of being a proficient clinician is quick recognition of management of ailments. A contributing factor to this is past experiences and pattern recognition. Being able to make connections between didactic knowledge in the clinical setting early on seems to provide pattern recognition that promote proficiency.

CHAPTER 7

Internship and Residency

— TIM'S EXPERIENCE —

When you are an intern, people address you as doctor. You have earned the right to make decisions in partnership with patients. You recognize the huge responsibility associated with your new position and at first you second guess yourself, overwhelmed with the magnitude of the responsibility. As an intern, you may feel intimidated, acutely aware of your lack of knowledge and experience. Sometimes fear enters your consciousness as you recognized the health and well-being of innocent people depend on your medical decision-making capacity. You learned in clerkship that you had a fiduciary responsibility to act in the best interest of the patient and you may doubt your ability to meet that standard.

Your initial decisions are made with caution, uncertainty, and trepidation. At first, you feel stupid because you ask the supervising resident the most simplistic questions. You check every decision by reviewing prior notes or pouring through the latest medical house staff manual. At the end of the day, you are drained of every ounce of emotional, mental, and physical energy. You would have collapsed but for your diet, exercise, and sleep routines. You fall asleep wondering how the system ever allowed you to become a doctor and whether anyone will die from your lack of experience and knowledge.

Soon, you realize the resident is checking every decision and order. Better yet, you see the patients are improving. The relationships you are building with the patients are warm, caring, and trustworthy. You begin to feel good about yourself in your new role as the doctor. The residents, fellows, and attending staff see your caring, giving manner, your curiosity to learn, and your comprehensive approach to patient care.

You develop a strong relationship with your resident—one built on open and honest communication, punctuality, thoroughness of work, and good ethics. Your reputation grows as you have a burning desire to learn more and to accept more responsibility. The team observes that you are accepting and responsive to critique and feedback. You do not have to be told to do anything twice.

You develop a trusting caring relationship with the support and nursing staff. Your emotional and social intelligence are paying dividends. You are identified as friendly, caring, approachable, smart, curious, and responsive to the needs of the patients and the staff. Everyone in the hospital feels better when you are the one on call. You can handle any situation.

INTERNSHIP AT THE MAYO CLINIC

As an intern at the Mayo Clinic, I felt the initial fear and uncertainty of being in the new role of doctor, but the supportive environment quickly helped me overcome my fears and uncertainty. The Mayo system was arranged to maximize learning in a setting where patient care was first and foremost.

As the intern, I was the first one to take a comprehensive history and physical examination of the patient. After my examination, the resident, and then the fellow completed their history and physical examination. Then we compared notes. The teaching was informative and positive; the exchange allowed me to develop a deeper understanding of the case. I would perform three to four new admissions, think through them on my own, discuss them with the resident and fellow, and then go home to read more about my cases. The next day, when presenting to the attending staff, I had been schooled well enough by the resident and fellow to seem relatively intelligent about the patient's clinical presentation, physical examination findings, and plan of care. The repetitive nature of this process helped me develop a foundation of knowledge in each rotation. In this type of environment, it is actually easy to learn.

My first rotation was cardiology, and in the end, I became a cardiologist. I chose cardiology for my career because of Dr. Tajik. He was my first consultant and became my life-long mentor. I was young and unaware that I was being tutored by one of the great minds in cardiology. The subsequent rotations were all great learning environments. The Mayo culture fosters learning and great patient care—a culture that resonates in the hallways of the clinic and the hospital. I essentially was spoon fed knowledge from the great minds in medicine throughout my three years of residency in internal medicine.

I realize that everyone cannot train at the Mayo Clinic. So wherever you train you must recreate that kind of environment. You must approach each day as a unique opportunity to learn. Each patient is an opportunity to integrate a history and physical examination. That integration should allow a synthesis of information to formulate a plan of care.

The advantage you have today that I didn't have is the rapid retrieval of information with PubMed and Google. After discussing the case with support staff you can go to the web and access the latest information on the problem you are tackling. Each patient is a unique opportunity to improve your history taking and physical examination skills, and your ability to synthesize information. You must see yourself as a medical sleuth. There is no limit to the learning you can achieve in a day if you are curious. In an odd way, the Internet allows you to train at the Mayo Clinic no matter where you are geographically. Your intellectual growth depends on your approach. Your only limitation will be yourself.

The growth and refinement of your emotional and social intelligence cannot be overstated. Look outside the box and evaluate every circumstance carefully to prevent poor decisions. This can best be illustrated by a Madison and Peppermint story. Madison and Peppermint, my two genius black labradors, are walking together. They walk in a circle with their heads down examining the ground, picking up a scent—sensing other creatures are invading their territory. They continue to walk in a circle, heads down, staying on the same path of the same scent.

The message here is that we are often caught up in a mad dash, heads down, following a well-trodden path. The failure to look around, pay attention to cues—verbal and non-verbal—prevents us from seeing the larger picture.

Perhaps if we looked up and perceived the larger reality, we would discover an alternative route that would take us to a more valuable spot.

Obey your instinct to look broadly at all situations. You must learn to practice due diligence when deciding how to approach your training. Listen to your own internal voice; acknowledge your internal reference points rather than just embracing the myriad external voices that may not have your best interest at heart. Your voice is not flawed, mistaken, or a distraction. Trust yourself and your instincts. Your instincts speak to your oldest and best neuronal connections. Listen to yourself.

By the same token, never be too proud to say, "I don't know." No one should expect you to know everything. "In training" means you're learning.

— ELIZABETH'S EXPERIENCE —

To be honest, I used to think the exorbitant amount of hours worked during residency was some hazing process to join an exclusive "old boys club" or fraternity. It is often difficult to appreciate the majesty of the great forest when one feels so lost roaming through the trees. It is only when you've had a chance to step back and reflect that you understand and truly appreciate the purpose of your journey through the forest. As Malcolm Gladwell alludes to in his book *Outliers*, many of the great figures of past and present, including Albert Einstein, Bill Gates, and Steve Jobs, achieved what they did because of the copious amounts of hours they invested in their trade. He alludes to the 10,000 hour principle: that people can become proficient in their chosen discipline if they practice it for 10,000 hours or more. Residency is an extension of this principle. We must put in the hours in order to solidify the medical knowledge we've acquired and make it second nature so we can treat patients in a timely and responsible manner and ensure the best outcome for them.

The novice interns who see their first case of a patient presenting to the emergency room with complaints of chest pain will automatically think "heart attack" and travel down the narrow road of ECG and cardiac enzymes and typically stop there. By the 100th evaluation for chest pain, a more experienced resident who has seen a wider range of pathologies causing chest discomfort will be able to automatically expand the differentials to not only cardiovascular causes (myocardial infarction, pericarditis, and aortic dissection, for example) but also pulmonary (pulmonary embolism), gastrointestinal (gastroesophageal reflux, pancreatitis with referred pain), and musculoskeletal (costochondritis). In addition to having more extensive differential diagnoses, the seasoned resident will also know how to ask appropriate questions and elicit physical exam findings that will narrow the list of differentials and tease out the true underlying etiology for the patient's chest discomfort.

In more procedural specialties such as surgery, the hours spent practicing become especially important. To become more proficient at performing any type of procedure or surgery, one has to actually do it. The eye-hand coordination required in surgery or performing procedures is a skillset that must be practiced manually and is not something that can be acquired by reading a book or manual, no matter how many hours spent reading it.

Another benefit of the extensive hours I experienced during residency that I would only later come to appreciate is that it heightened my sense of empathy. After a busy 24-hour shift of call, I was fatigued beyond words, ached, and was famished. I had inadvertently skipped lunch and dinner the day before due to constant admissions and patient care issues, and was nauseous from sleep deprivation. When I was rounding on my patients in the morning, I came by to check on a patient whom I had admitted the evening before. He had Non-Hodgkin's lymphoma—a cancer of the lymphatic system—and had completed a round of chemotherapy that left him immunosuppressed with mucositis, an inflammatory condition that resulted in the multiple painful sores and ulcerations in his mouth. Because of the sores and chemotherapy, he had lost his appetite and had not eaten for days, which resulted in dehydration and acute kidney injury.

The cancer ravaged his body, causing him to be chronically fatigued while his abdomen constantly ached. Despite all of this, when I walked into his room that morning, he greeted me with the most incredible smile. "Doc, you look worse than me!" he exclaimed. This instantly made me laugh and I told him I agreed. Even with the discomfort he had and weakness he felt, he still took the time that morning to ask me how the rest of my call night was and if I ever got to sleep or eat. "You asked me all those questions when you admitted me last night, it's only fair I ask you the same questions!" he said.

Here we were, both tired and aching, sleep and food deprived, yet I knew my discomfort would end when I got home and had a good night's sleep and dinner. His, however, would persist so long as the cancer was there and he had to go through chemotherapy. During the course of my residency, I had the opportunity to meet so many patients of all diversities, personalities, and ailments. From each and every patient I had the honor of caring for, I learned so much about medical pathology, but more importantly about humanity.

It was during my residency that I had the opportunity to work with some incredible attending physicians who took the time to teach and encourage more in-depth analysis of patients' medical problems and treatment plans. My advice to those going through training is not to shy away from attending's who have a reputation of being "tough." If that attending is considered tough because he or she is malicious, does not teach, and makes learning difficult, then that's another matter. However, if an attending earns a reputation as being "tough" because he or she challenges the residents to think more critically, investigate their patient's illness more thoroughly, and push their limits intellectually, embrace the opportunity to work with that attending. You may be tired from the longer hours you'll have to work to know your patients and often frustrated from the constant barrage of questions about your patient's presentation, or management, from this critical attending. However, when all is said and done and you look back at your training, you'll realize your higher level of proficiency is because the tough attending challenged and taught you.

In my residency, there was such an attending who was a nephrologist by specialty and who was scheduled to do inpatient wards with medicine residents various months through the year. During the months he was on, many of the residents who were assigned to him would often groan, knowing they a tough month ahead of them. It was during my second year of residency that I had a ward month with him. The first day of that month was daunting as he walked in and gave a stern look to me and my fellow interns, followed by a quick lecture about his expectations of us while rotating with him that month. This began a whirlwind month of extrapolating minute details from patients about their medical complaints and history, obtaining countless numbers of documents from outside hospitals and dialysis centers, and constantly reading articles available on PubMed to substantiate our medical decisions.

You could not simply admit a noncompliant patient for "volume overload secondary to missed dialysis session." During your presentation of this patient, you had to not only know what days the patient usually received dialysis and the dialysis site (tunnel line, AV fistula, etc.), but you also had to obtain the records from their dialysis center so you had information about the amount of volume they typically removed during each dialysis session, the electrolytes and dialysis solution used for the dialysis, and their dry weight. From this information, you might find out that perhaps their volume overload was not from the kidney disease but some other patho-logical process in the body that you may have missed if you had not done a thorough investigation. The attending constantly asked what "evidence" we had to substantiate our medical decisions and why we picked certain therapies, or performed the test we did, or decided on the diagnosis we did. His questions forced us to go back to the patient to extract more informa-tion through history or physical exam and research available information from the medical literature on the topic.

Through the hard work, there was great satisfaction in seeing his face break out in a smile when we brought him a handful of literature to support our decisions, or when we knew a slight bit more about the patient's history than he did. One great thing about him was that he led by example. He read up on the patients' history and ailments and obtained information from the dialysis centers well before we ever did. As hard as we worked, he worked harder to know the patients and what was going on with them. He did not take satisfaction in our failures. Instead, he took delight in our accomplishments, whether it a tidbit about our patient's history that he was not able to get on his own, or coming up with diagnoses that he had not thought of, or even better, the correct diagnosis!

During wards with him, we looked beyond the superficial and investigated deeper. We avoided unnecessary testing and treatments if there was no substantial evidence for it based on the patient's clinical presentation. By the end of the rotation, the trust and approval I gained from this attending was rewarding, and the increased proficiency and astuteness I ascertained, as a physician, was priceless. Tough love has the potential to be a great learning tool.

CHAPTER 8

Fellowship Training

— TIM'S EXPERIENCE —

The choice of specialized medical or surgical training is usually easy. Those who choose advanced training typically are driven by their quest for a deeper understanding of an area of medicine. For me, there was no question: I knew I wanted to pursue my passion, which was cardiology.

The opportunity for advanced training in any area is exciting when you are pursuing a passion—a field of medicine that instills pure joy in your heart. I consider myself lucky because I get a paycheck and I have never "worked." My fellowship years were a special time because I was developing an expertise in a field I loved and, most important, my wife and I had our two boys, TJ and Zachary.

I was fortunate to be at the Mayo Clinic in Rochester, Minnesota. As I rotated through the different areas of cardiac catheterization, echocardiography, nuclear medicine, electrophysiology, coronary care unit, and outpatient cardiology, I was learning cardiac catheterization from David Holmes, nuclear cardiology from Ray Gibbons, echocardiography from Jamil Tajik and Jim Seward, and many more giants in the field. I enjoyed each area immensely as I was talking with the people who wrote the book in the particular area I was rotating through that month. This experience increased my competence across a broad and vast array of issues in cardiology.

The cardiac catheterization laboratory was intellectually stimulating, challenging, and intimidating. The approach to coronary artery disease and hemodynamics was intriguing and fun. The staff members in the cardiac catheterization lab at Mayo Clinic–Rochester were all masters in the field of cardiac cath and outstanding, dedicated teachers. I had been an athlete and had played Division 1 college basketball, which improved my eye–hand coordination. College sports also gave me thick skin and mental toughness. I was certain these attributes would serve me well in the catheterization laboratory, where it is important to maintain composure when confronted with patients who are critically ill—situations where on-the-spot thinking and immediate reactions can determine a patient's fate.

Then I met David Holmes, the director of the cardiac catheterization laboratory. He was quite intimidating and could have held his own with any college basketball coach. He was critical and constantly testing the fellows' internal fabric, toughness, and ability to withstand the stress of the cath lab. I despised him during my rotation, and tried to scrub in with Dennis or John Breshahan, brothers who not only were talented cath doctors, but had played college basketball, which gave us something to bond over. Over time, I became more comfortable working with Dr. Holmes. He was superb at performing complex procedures and I learned to appreciate his skills.

Another notable teacher in the cath lab who influenced me during training was Rick Nishamura. Rick was a brilliant thinker and enthusiastic about cardiology. He was a master of hemodynamics in the cath lab and used his excellence there and in echo lab hemodynamics to teach the fellows.

During my fellowship, I learned from many outstanding doctors, including A. Jamil Tajik and James Seward, who are known around the world for their expertise in echocardiography, and Ray Gibbons, my teacher in nuclear cardiology, who was a truly insightful, gifted teacher. How lucky I was to have crossed paths with these great teachers who have remained my friends over the years.

Fellowship was an amazing time and experience and I learned to find a good balance between family and work—which brings me back to essentialism: You must define the essentials in your life and stay committed to them.

During this time I experienced the joy of my two boys being born. TJ, our first, was constantly on the go. I remember being on call for 24 hours in a very busy cardiac care unit (CCU) at St. Mary's Hospital and coming home to an exhausted Barb, who had been "on call" with TJ. As I entered the house, she said, "Your turn." Zachary was born soon after. He decided, in utero, to be the polar opposite of TJ. He was shy, introverted, sweet and quiet.

As you consider fellowship training, make it as rewarding and as enjoyable as possible. Learn all you can while making time for family and friends. Be sure to network during fellowship—reach out to find the work opportunity that is right for you and your family. The more contacts you have the better. You must find a practice that has similar ideology to your own in terms of work and life balance.

The landscape of medicine has changed and the corporatization of medicine has made it more difficult to find opportunities that understand your needs. Most of these organizations are bottom line balance sheet factories and they often see you as the factory worker. Subsequent chapters will give you some insights into the state of medicine today. As you begin to understand the impact of corporate medicine on physicians, nurses, NPs, and PAs, you will be better prepared to meet the future.

— ELIZABETH'S EXPERIENCE —

The teachers you encounter during your residency can have a significant impact on your career choices. By teachers, I mean not only attending physicians, but also the fellows and upper residents who through their guidance and tutorship make you appreciate and understand topics that you encounter during your rotations.

Unlike Tim, I did not immediately know I wanted to go into cardiology at the beginning of training. Cardiology, at first, seemed like such an intimidating specialty. The squiggles and lines of the ECG were like a foreign language that needed translating. The shadows and flashes of bright colors of the echo images were like artworks that only true art connoisseurs knew the meaning behind. The cath lab was a place where lightening quick decisions were made. During my ward rotation as an intern, I was fortunate enough to have a smart and quick-witted resident as my senior. He knew from day one of his medical career that he wanted to become a cardiologist and had an abundance of cardiology knowledge beyond what most second-year residents have. He helped me makes sense of the squiggles and lines and gain a deeper understanding behind those ECG tracings.

During my rotation on the CCU and cardiology consults, I was blessed to work with cardiology fellows who took the time to teach and help me understand echocardiographic images, myocardial perfusion images, and cardiac catheterizations. Through their guidance, cardiology was no longer intimidating, and became much more enjoyable as I slowly figured out the meaning behind the tracings and hemodynamics behind the echoes and heart catheterizations. It was through the encouragement and mentor-ship provided by my upper residents and cardiology fellows that I became interested in a specialty I would have otherwise not even considered.

Now, as a fellow, I often think about those great mentors of my past who taught me so much and I try to do the same for the residents who rotate through cardiology with me. With changes in medical policies, there seems to be a never-ending number of logistical and social issues that can make patient care overwhelming. The irony of electronic medical record (EMR) is that it's supposed to make document-keeping more efficient, yet it's gen-erated more work with the copious amounts of clicks and typing you must do to satisfy quality of care measures, or even do a "simple" history and physical document. Though the impact of the copious amount "electronic work" on medical training and education has not been objectively evaluated in studies, many trainees will likely agree that it takes out a substantial amount of their day typing notes and checking boxes that could have been spent talking to patients or studying.

With this in mind, a typical workday in the cardiac care unit, for example, is busy, and there don't seem to be enough hours to complete what you want to get accomplished, let alone sit down and teach residents. Yet it is important to do so, since they are future healthcare practitioners and what they learn during their training is what they carry through during their own practice.

AT THE FOUNDATION

This practice of teaching those under our tutelage is a tradition that's the core basis of medical training. Kenneth Ludmerer, in his book *Let Me Heal*, does a beautiful job of chronicling the evolution of medical training from its early days of unstructured apprenticeship to the development of the ACGME-structured medical training programs of residency and fellowship that we now have today. It helps us appreciate our forefathers of medicine who realized the importance of education and in particular *structured* clinical education on which to build a foundation for competent future physicians.

There was an emphasis by the attendings on spending time talking to the patients and doing a thorough exam to produce comprehensive differential diagnoses. Granted, our healthcare predecessors had much less paperwork demands and patient load than is the case today, but it does not take away the importance of eliciting a good history and physical exam. Today, as soon as a patient walks through the ER door and says he has chest pain, the doctor orders cardiac enzymes, ECG, chest radiographs, and possibly a chest CT or echocardiogram. When a patient presents with syncope, a head CT, ECG, and echocardiogram is immediately ordered before thought is given to getting a good history and physical examination.

During my fellowship, I was fortunate enough to cross paths with Tim Paterick, who became my great mentor and friend. He not only took the time to educate those around him, but also encourages critical thinking and deeper understanding of patients as well as cardiac pathophysiology. He took the time to do a thorough physical examination and correlate it with echocardiographic findings rather than vice versa. He welcomed questions and challenges from the fellows and residents. He smiled warmly when we were right because he took joy in watching our knowledge grow before his eyes. He was a great leader by example. He would take on more work, whether in the echo lab or in CCU, if it meant more time at the patient bedside teaching us physical exam findings or giving formal didactics. For those going through any type of residency or fellowship in any kind of subspecialty, I hope you have the opportunity to have a mentor like Dr. Paterick, because it will make your training experience all the more rewarding.

Part Three

Going Out to Practice

CHAPTER 9

Searching for the "Ideal" Professional Job

You have worked hard to earn your medical degree and your specialty training. Now it is equally important to give the same level of effort and thought to finding your ideal professional job opportunity.

A lack of critical analysis by physicians seeking employment may reflect one of the manifestations of a pervasive optimist. Most of us perceive the world as more benign than it really is, our own attributes as more favorable than they truly are, and the goals we adopt as more achievable than they are likely to be. We tend to exaggerate our ability to forecast the future, which fosters optimistic overconfidence. In terms of its consequences for decisions, in particular employment decisions, this optimistic bias may be a significant cognitive bias and may have inherent costs. This can create real risks.

Physicians have been educated in a healthcare paradigm that is reactive, responding to diseases rather than preventing their development. Physicians seeking employment should not apply this reactive paradigm to their job search. They must be relentless and precise in their search for an organization that creates and maintains a work environment that enables the staff to have a healthy balance between work and personal responsibilities, such as family, friends, and community. This work-life balance is vital to physical, mental, emotional and family health. Success in life must be defined beyond career.

Your understanding of the complexity of a physician's life should cause you to carefully consider how you will approach your future. What do you need to know? *Due diligence* refers to the care a reasonable person should take before entering into an agreement or transaction with another party.

Due diligence is essential for healthcare providers because in the new business model of medicine, physicians are being employed by large healthcare organizations that require their employed physicians to sign legally binding employment contracts.

This chapter provides guidance for physicians who are planning to enter into a contractual relationship to become professional employees of a large healthcare organization such as a hospital, medical group, ACO, or Medical Home. While the employment contracts used by some of these large organizations appropriately balance the interests of both parties, many organizations may use a contract that greatly favors the organization, and seriously disadvantages the individual physician employee. So it is extremely important in your quest for your ideal professional opportunity to understand the implications of any employment contract prior to signing it.

Physicians would be wise to seek expertise through an employment coach to become educated about marketplace salaries; health, dental, disability, and malpractice insurance; retirement benefits; savings plans; and the legal ramifications of their employment agreement. Additional considerations include paid time off, cafeteria plans setting aside pretax dollars for items not covered by insurance, annual educational benefits, and professional fees and dues. This proactive approach to seeking employment will prevent postemployment regret and despair.

The dilemma facing physicians today, in an era of employed physicians, is frequently similar to David vs. Goliath! Use the metaphorical stone of due diligence to arm yourself with knowledge.

Before you sign, ask yourself: Have all questions regarding the contract been carefully considered? Are there more questions than answers? Identify the issues before signing the contract or commencing work. The time to fully understand the contractual relationship nuances is before starting employment. Consult an expert in contracts. Make a wise investment of your time and money: the upfront costs may avoid much higher costs and major frustrations in the future.

Here are some considerations as you find your ideal job.

SALARY

Will your salary be consistent with your training? Will your salary be consistent with your experience level? Will your salary be consistent with similar specialists' salaries in your geographic area? Is there a signing bonus? Depending on your qualifications and the needs of the organization, this could be a significant benefit.

The variables that influence physician salary include the location and needs of the employer organization, specialty training of the physician, and board certification. When starting a new practice, a base salary is usually guaranteed for the first two or three years. A base salary plus an incentive/bonus amount based on a productivity formula determine subsequent salary. The issues relating to productivity income can be complex. Productivity may be calculated from individual physician billings, but is more likely calculated from actual collections from those billings. The distinction is important because collections on billings are determined by payer mix of the billings, contracts negotiated by the organization, and the effectiveness of the billing/collection department. Additional variables that affect the physician's salary include quality metrics and patient satisfaction surveys.

Special attention should be paid to the signing bonus, as it may have tax implications and under some circumstances must be repaid. Also, be aware that organizations expect physicians' professional skills to be used exclusively for the benefit of the organization and any outside income is simply credited as additional productivity in the income distribution formula. Outside income may include moonlighting, honoraria for speaking engagements, medical-legal review, insurance claims review, and pharmaceutical-sponsored activities.

INSURANCE

Health: Will you and your family be adequately covered?

Disability: Who will pay the bills if you are suddenly disabled?

Life: Who will provide for your family in the event of your premature death?

Malpractice: What professional liability coverage is provided? Who makes the decisions regarding resolving claims?

Insurance considerations include health, dental, life, disability, and medical malpractice. Ideally, the employer should provide these insurance benefits, and health and dental insurance should include the physician and his or her family. The co-pays and deductibles must be reasonable and it is important to identify costs for going outside the network.

Life insurance is an important part of providing financial security for your family. Term life insurance is usually the best value, and ideally, if you terminate your employment, the policy will go with you if you pay the premiums. Disability insurance is crucial for physicians with young families. The present movement is for employers to not provide disability insurance, or to provide a limited benefit. If insufficient life or disability coverage is provided, strong consideration should be given to purchasing a private policy.

Malpractice insurance is essential and must be adequate based on the specialty. If the policy is not "occurrence-based," then tail coverage—covering claims after the physician leaves the practice—is essential and should be provided by the employer. Additionally, it is important for physicians to be involved in the manner in which claims are handled. In some states, settlement could affect physician licensure, so the physician has his or her reputation and licensure at risk.

RETIREMENT BENEFITS

Do you have a plan for retirement? Does the contract support your plan? Retirement plans vary, but are typically defined contributions plans (401k) rather than defined benefit (pension) plans. Contribution amounts are typically a percentage of your annual salary. Ideally, the employer will match your contribution. You should seek immediate vesting and be allowed to control how your retirement funds are invested.

PAID LEAVE

Paid time off is important and includes vacation days, sick days, family leave, holidays, time for continuing medical education, and personal days. Paid time off should be defined in the contract. Determine whether accumulated leave is lost if it is not used annually.

PROFESSIONAL EXPENSES

Professional expenses that should be paid by the organization include state license fee, DEA fee, hospital staff dues, and costs of continuing medical education, including travel expenses. Organizations may also pay for national, state, and county medical societies.

MOVING EXPENSES

Depending on the distance required, moving expenses might be significant. It is standard for employers to pay a reasonable stipend for moving expenses. The employment agreement should define the amount of reimbursement and any restrictions as to when the move occurs, who does the moving, and the policy on pay back if there is a contract termination.

THE RESTRICTIVE COVENANT

Restrictive covenants are common in employment contracts, so you need to learn to identify and understand the future limitations imposed on you by any restrictive covenant in your contract. A restrictive covenant is a clause within a contract that stipulates the limitations of where you may practice or provide services once you leave your current employer or medical group. Restrictive covenants preclude competition within a certain geographical area for a certain time. Although there is variance among states, restrictive covenants are typically enforceable if considered reasonable in the eyes of the law. Additional restriction might include the prohibition of solicitation of patients and co-workers.

These restrictions must be understood, as they may be professionally, financially, and personally disadvantageous if you terminate employment and decide to contest the restrictive covenant. The following are a few prerequisites for restrictive covenants to be enforceable. The employer must:

- Have a protected interest in justifying the restriction on the activity of the employee.
- Provide a reasonable time limit for the restriction.
- Provide a reasonable territorial limit for the restriction.
- Have a restriction that is not oppressive to the employee or contrary to public policy.

Learn everything about any restrictive covenants before you sign a contract.

TERMINATION

Can you be terminated *without* good cause? Can you be terminated *with* good cause? How long do benefits continue upon termination? How is pay determined during the notice period?

Termination is possible and you must at least consider and plan for this possibility. If it does occur, you will wish you had engaged legal representation prior to employment. Understanding the actions and omissions that trigger termination are important so one can plan to avoid them. If possible, avoid contracts that include termination without cause. For termination with cause, the contract should clearly delineate the causes that trigger termination. Important components of the termination policy are the termination notice period and whether the time period is equal for both employer- and employee-instigated termination, by whom and how termination is determined, length of time benefits continue, and how income is determined during the notice period. Most contracts will outline termination for "material breaches," such as loss of medical license, substance abuse, and criminal acts.

LEGAL FEES

Many organizations require the employee to pay the legal fees of the organization if a legal dispute arises. This is a quote from an employment agreement emphasizing this point:

> *"The parties agree that damages will not sufficiently compensate the Organization for a breach of a Restrictive Covenant, and that in the event of an actual or threatened breach of the Restrictive Covenant, the Organization shall have the right to petition the court of jurisdiction for injunctive relief or for other equitable relief, in addition to all other remedies allowed by law. In the event the Organization is successful in a lawsuit enforcing the provisions of this agreement the Employee, in addition to all other remedies, the Organization shall be entitled to recover all costs of litigation, including reasonable attorney's fees, from the Employee."*

Note the agreement does not state that the employee shall be entitled to recover all costs of litigation, including reasonable attorney's fees, from the organization in the event the employee prevails in the legal dispute. These issues must be critically analyzed before any contract is signed, as the legal process at the time of terminating employment can cause the employee to endure enormous financial and emotional debt.

EMPLOYEE APPROACH TO EMPLOYMENT

Start early to identify employment opportunities. Understand the contract, policies, procedures, and culture of the organization. The contract is your lens into the culture of the organization. Identify how the organization has treated physicians historically. Contract law governs the legal aspects of a contract. Most physician contracts are written, but some may be verbal, as well. The failure to adhere to the promises made in these written or verbal contracts is considered a breach. Contract law provides legal remedies for the party adversely affected by the breach. An obligation to fulfill the contract exists, and the edicts of contract law will determine the penalty for failure to do so.

It is important to seek expertise to help you understand the nuisances of the contract and how to negotiate a fair contract with symmetry. Remember that contracts are negotiable. Physicians traditionally have not been educated in business and law, and frequently feel uncomfortable negotiating—all the more reason to seek expertise when confronting these complex employment issues. Negotiate everything upfront because once the contract is signed, it's game over.

GENERAL COMPONENTS OF AN "IDEAL" PROFESSIONAL JOB

Work-Life Balance: Search for an organization that creates and maintains a work environment that enables its staff to have a healthy balance between work and personal responsibilities, such as family, friends, recreation, reflection, community activities. Work-Life balance does not mean an equal balance. This work-life balance in your life is vital for good physical, mental, emotional, and spiritual health. Identifying the right work place requires networking, asking colleagues, and when visiting the site paying attention to all verbal and non-verbal ques. Identify if people seem happy and sincere, or if responses are strained and robotic. It is imperative that you pay attention to the culture of the work environment. While visiting ask people for phone numbers for follow up calls. You're looking for a good fit for you.

— ELIZABETH'S CORNER —

The completion of residency or fellowship is an exciting time. You are finally an autonomous practicing physician! After years of medical school combined with residency and possible fellowship, it is hard to not ecstatically and blindly look at the proverbial "light at the end of tunnel" and forget that that "light" could very well be an oncoming train.

After years of working countless hours at the average annual salary equivalency of the higher range for an administrative assistant, many graduating residents and fellows are happy to finally go out and practice on their own, having some control over their hours at a pay grade that's seems relatively significant compared to their trainee salary. Also, given the expensive tuition of medical school training with an average debt of $250,000, many newly graduated trainees are in debt with student loans. These factors, in conjunction with sheer inexperience at contractual negotiations, unfortunately result in the mistake of settling for subpar contract agreements. The pitfalls in the contract come to light over time, as the individual finds him or herself in an unsatisfactory work environment or situation.

Although there are no guarantees in life, it's important to arm yourself with as much knowledge as possible when searching for your ideal medical practice, whether it is a private medical group or a hospital conglomerate.

As you start the job search, take time for introspection. Decide what your ideal job is and whether it's possible based on the circumstances you're in. Those who are single may have more freedom in terms of location or type of work available (i.e., locums tenens in which you travel and work as needed), while their counterparts with a family may be slightly more restricted in options. Questions to think about include:

- Do you prefer mostly outpatient or inpatient type of settings or vice versa?
- Is the trade-off of higher patient census or more calls worth the higher salary?
- What are your ultimate goals? Work hard and retire early or work in moderation until retirement?

- Do you enjoy teaching? Research? If yes, then you would prefer to be in an academic setting. If no, then you may enjoy medical practice in a private setting.

Once you've made a list of your personal goals, the ideal job, and possible locations, take the information provided in this chapter and make a check list of each of the items discussed and ensure that the questions are addressed in each job interview you go on. Similar to the process you underwent as you made your decisions for ranking medical schools and residency/fellowship, immediately fill out this check list after each job interview and make notes of the pros and cons of each job location.

Use as many resources as possible to learn about the current group or hospital to understand the politics and dynamics you'll have to work in on a daily basis. As much as we would like to say "work is work" and think that we can somehow separate it from our personal lives, in reality it is very hard to do, especially if work ends up making up half of your day. So invest the time it takes to analyze your future workplace as well as the individual components of your contract to ensure that you are getting a secure and fair deal. Invest in a lawyer if you don't fully understand the legal jargon. The money and time you invest in thoroughly exploring your job options and contract will be worth the headache and heartache you can avoid in the future.

CHAPTER 10

Gaining Perspective in a Chaotic World

Most physicians are just trying to do the best they can in situations where they are seeing too many patients, in too little time, and attempting to meet unrealistic RVU goals to maintain their salary. When demand exceeds capacity, physicians make expedient choices that get them through the day, but take an emotional and physical toll over time. The toll can result in suboptimal clinical decisions, too little sleep, a sedentary lifestyle, and fast food on the run, coffee to fuel up, and sleeping pills to calm down. Physicians often return home from the fast and furious pace of work feeling exhausted and seeing their family not as a source of joy, but as another demand in an already-overburdened life.

Smartphone apps, to do lists, pagers, e-mail, phone messages, and pop-up reminders are all designed to help physicians manage time more efficiently and to be more productive for the organization. There is pride in the ability to multitask and work long hours—it's a badge of honor. The 24/7 schedules describe a world where work never ends. Physicians have been indoctrinated to believe words like *obsessed*, *crazed*, and *overwhelmed* describe our everyday life rather than an insane existence. Physicians feeling forever stressed for time assume they have no choice but to cram as much as possible into every day to survive.

What has gone wrong? Why are physicians living in a state of chaos? In his book *The Signal and the Noise: Why Most Predictions Fail—but Some Don't*, Nate Silver examines the world of predictions, investigating how we can distinguish a true signal from the noise of ever-increasing data. He examines chaos theory across many domains to help understand the impact of small changes in a dynamic system. The application of chaos theory to the healthcare model will give us insight into the reasons healthcare delivery is failing, why physicians are burning out, and what we can do about it.

THE THEORY BEHIND CHAOS

Chaos theory applies to systems in which each of two properties exist: 1) the system is dynamic, meaning the behavior at one point in time influences behavior in the future, and 2) the system is nonlinear, meaning change results in exponential rather than additive relationship—akin to the stock market. The intersection of a dynamic system with exponential change can result in a real mess: as it has in today's healthcare delivery system.

The most basic tenet of chaos theory is that small changes in initial conditions produce large and unexpected divergence in outcomes. Certain outcomes of "system change" are hard to predict. The problem begins when there are the inevitable inaccuracies in our assumptions. For example, let's say we want to compute 5+5 but accidently key in 6 for the second entry. We have an outcome of 11 rather than 10. We are wrong, but not by much because addition is a linear function that is forgiving.

Alternatively, in dynamic systems like healthcare, exponential functions extract significant punishment when there are inaccuracies in our assumptions. If instead of calculating 5^3 (125) calculate 5^4 (625), we have missed our end point by 500%! This inaccuracy explodes if the system is dynamic and this output feeds into the next input algorithm. Thus our small, trivial mistake results in a much greater mistake.

Human beings are the epitome of a dynamic system with nonlinear behaviors that are highly vulnerable to inaccuracies in prediction. There are medical models were prediction has failed, often at a cost to society. In 2005, an article evaluated the positive findings in peer-reviewed articles: descriptions of successful predictions of medical hypotheses carried out in laboratory experiments where two-thirds of the findings could not be replicated. This reinforces the notion that our predictive models are flawed. Why? Because the smaller the study, the less likely the research findings are to be true; the smaller the effects, the less likely the research findings are to be true; the greater the financial interests, the less likely the research findings are to be true.

We must return to the paradigm of considering new insights null and void without compelling evidence. Add to this the fact that we are exploding with new information with the introduction of the Internet. The quantity of information is increasing by 2.5 quintillion bytes per day, but the amount of useful information in this exploding data set is unknown. Most of this information is noise, and the noise is increasing faster than the truth. There are so many hypotheses to test, so much data to mine, but a relatively small amount of meaningful, useful information.

Complex systems like the World Wide Web can reproduce a mistake many times over. It may not fail as many times as a simple system, but when its fails, the result has exponential impact. This incredible, rapid, and efficient information machine has the potential to spread bad ideas and information. This should cause us to pause and reflect on what information we are putting into our models, as we have so much noise we cannot identify the objective truths we need to use to have accurate prediction models.

The illusions of validity and skill are supported by a powerful professional culture. People can maintain an unshakeable faith in any proposition, however absurd, when a community of like-minded believers sustains them. Given the professional culture of the medical community, it is not surprising that large numbers of individuals in the world believe themselves to be the chosen few who can lead the rest.

STATISTICAL ILLITERACY

Because we are influenced by stories, we must remember they represent individual, anecdotal events that may make an impression upon us, but may not represent the experience of the population. Statistics can help put anecdotal messages into a larger context. Health literacy—understanding statistics about the risks and benefits of therapy—allows us to grasp the scientific data and make a more considered choice than using narratives in isolation.

For example, we all have a well-marketed narrative by the drug companies about the impact of high cholesterol on our health. A common notion is that taking a statin will reduce your risk of a heart attack by 30% over the next 10 years. Why would anyone not take a statin? Let's look into the facts.

There is an algorithm that allows a calculation of your risk for a heart attack over 10 years. This algorithm considers age, sex, total cholesterol, good cholesterol (HDL), blood pressure, smoking status, family history, and medications. Let's assume the risk identified is 1%. This means 1 of 100 people with this risk will have a heart attack over the next 10 years. So what does it mean that a statin will reduce one's risk of a heart attack by 30% over the next 10 years?

Let's become statistically literate. Your 1% risk means you have a 1 in 100 chance of a heart attack. This implies 3 in 300 will have a heart attack. The statin treatment reduces the risk by 30%. The 300 patients with a 1% risk would suggest three heart attacks without statin treatment. Thus, treating all 300 patients would prevent one heart attack (30% or 1/3 of a total of 3 people who would have a heart attack). The other two patients would have a heart attack despite taking the statin. The remaining 297 patients would not have a heart attack without the medication, but would incur the expense and the risk of side effects. This 300 represents the number needed to treat in order to help one person. This data can be framed in a positive narrative—a statin will reduce a heart attack by 30%—or in a negative narrative—300 people need to be treated to help one person.

There is a distinct lack of statistical literacy being applied to clinical scenarios. Bayes theorem allows clinicians to determine the probability that a hypothesis is true if some event has occurred. Let's reinforce this important concept by looking at a simple model:

BREAST CANCER AMONG WOMEN IN THEIR 40S

- The chance a women in her 40s will develop breast cancer is 1.4% (14/1000)
- A mammogram will be a false positive about 10% of the time.
- If breast cancer is present, the mammogram detects it 75% of the time.

Initially, these statistics paint a negative picture. But if you apply Bayes theorem, you will come to a different conclusion: the chance that a women in her 40s with a positive mammogram has breast cancer is 10%; the false positives dominate the calculus because the prevalence is 1.4%. Testing predictive models must be applied to get past unproven narratives and illusions, as the breast cancer example demonstrates.

TECHNOLOGY AND DECISION MAKING

The business medical models and evolving technology and marketing have overtaken the critical thought necessary for considered medical decisions. Let me share a clinical scenario that substantiates the impact of technology on medical decision-making.

A 50-year-old active, lean attorney came in for a second opinion. His 49th birthday present from his wife had been a computed tomography scan of his heart. The calcium score was high and the rollercoaster ride began. A A cardiac angiogram was performed and four stents were placed without stress testing and in a setting of no symptoms. (He had been working out on an elliptical for 45 minutes a day, five days per week.) He was started on a drug regiment including a statin, beta blocker, aspirin, and Plavix.

At the initial consultation for the second opinion, the patient was fatigued, had muscle aches that prevented any exercise, was unable to sustain an erection, was depressed, and fearful a stent would "clot off"—all because of a wife who responded to an advertisement and a physician who was practicing in chaos. This problem of inappropriate use or overuse of medical procedures is rampant as the physicians, hospitals, and device industry are all aligned and incentivized to do more.

The models and paradigms that have been forced upon physicians were never adequately tested and the exponential fluctuations that have occurred in healthcare as a result of these changes have resulted in a healthcare crisis. The physician work place is dynamic and nonlinear. There have been constant shakeups over the past 40 years, including managed care models, employee status, and business models of medicine run by corporate teams, Affordable Care Act changing reimbursement, changing care paradigms with nurse practitioners, physician assistants, electronic medical records, mandated schedules, and RVU expectations.

The most recent perturbation was the introduction of ICD–10 into the reporting world of physicians in October 2015. This new code set increased the number of reporting codes from about 13,600 to 69,000 and it represents a dramatic increase in reporting detail and granularity. In this context, granularity is defined as a deeper level of detail. This increasing complexity in coding has potential for exponential increase in errors and loss of physician time spent with patients.

No true hypothesis testing was performed to identify whether any of these "small" changes with exponential affects would be successful in the care of patients. These alterations have led to physicians running on a hedonic treadmill resulting in physician anger, fear, anxiety, resentfulness, depression, exhaustion, and hopelessness.

BACK TO THE ESSENTIALS

The answer to complex problems is simplification—distillation to essential components that are manageable and predictable. We have wandered a long way down a misguided path of medical care with layers of confusing bureaucracy. Physicians must understand the dynamic medical systems in the new business model of medicine are nonlinear and running out of control. They must be proactive and unify to protect patients and their own professionalism.

The baseball team cannot play without the players and the healthcare system cannot function without physicians. The future of our society's health depends on concerted efforts by physicians to ensure patient-centered models. The exponential ramifications of untested changes in the delivery of healthcare must be stopped. Simplification requires fewer players and simpler models that prioritize patient care.

CHAPTER 11

Making Choices: The Libby Zion Case

Resident duty hours have been a point of debate for many years. The Libby Zion case precipitated the movement to restrict and limit work hours for residents because resident fatigue was thought to be the culprit for medical error. However, it's important to ask whether this is truly the only conclusion to be drawn from the case.

This case occurred with an intern and resident providing the patient care, but could apply to NPCs. As you read this chapter, identify yourself as the NP, PA, intern, or resident involved in the described scenario.

Libby Zion was an 18-year-old college student admitted by a New York City hospital in 1984 with a fever and an earache. Six hours after admission, she was dead. Primarily an ER resident and an intern administered the medical care she received—restraints and Demerol. An attending physician did not see Libby. Her father, Sidney Zion, a *New York Times* journalist, requested an investigation into his daughter's death, and a grand jury investigation was convened.

The grand jury brought no criminal charges, but instead indicted a medical education system that allowed overtired, unsupervised residents and interns to treat a seriously ill patient with only sedatives and restraints. Among the grand jury's recommendations were:

1. Hospitals should staff emergency departments with physicians who have at least three years of training and who are specifically qualified to evaluate patients on an emergent basis;
2. Junior residents and interns should be supervised by attending physicians at all times; and

3. The New York Department of Health should promulgate regulations limiting the number of hours worked by interns and residents in teaching hospitals. The implication being that a tired resident and intern had made decisions that prevented an unfortunate outcome.

In response to the grand jury recommendations, the New York State Health Department appointed an ad hoc advising committee—the Bell Commission—to make specific proposals to implement the grand jury's recommendations. The committee received testimony from representatives of several of the most influential organizations responsible for graduate medical education, including the American College of Physicians and the American Medical Association. The majority of witnesses who testified before the Bell Commission opposed the imposition of any quantitative restriction on resident hours and proffered several reasons for leaving the existing on-call schedule intact:

1. Decision-making and execution of complex technical tasks under the duress of extreme fatigue are the *sine qua non* of medical practice. According to the Ad Hoc Advisory Committee testimony of F. Davidoff, American College of Physicians: "It would be unrealistic to expect residents to absorb the realities of caring for their equally fragile and needy patients if their working hours were fixed according to an arbitrary schedule, however well intended."
2. Continuity of care requires that the same resident who admits or operates on a patient should follow the patient through his or her illness, meaning the resident must not relinquish the case to another physician even after 24 hours. According to the Ad Hoc Advisory Committee testimony of J. Albers, MD, of the American Medical Association: "The care of my patients is enhanced when the physician who initially evaluated them after admission to the hospital cares for them for an extended period of time."
3. The cost of hiring additional nurses, lab personnel, and transport personnel would be prohibitive.

The Bell Commission issued its recommendations, which included the following proposal:

> "Individual residents who have direct patient care responsibilities in areas other than the ED shall have a scheduled work

week which will not exceed an average of 80 hours per week over a four-week period, and should not be scheduled to work as a matter of course more than 24 consecutive hours with one 24-hour period of non-working time per week. Teaching hospitals will develop specific standards dealing with schedules and limits of responsibility of individual residents during consecutive working hours, including responsibility for evaluation of new patients. This recommendation applies to anesthesiology, family practice, medical, surgical, obstetrical, pediatric, or other services which have a high numbers of acute ill patients" (Working Conditions of Residents and the Issue of Ancillary Help, in Ad Hoc Advisory Committee).

In 1989, the New York State Health Department incorporated these regulations into its hospital code. The revised regulations provided that: 1) residents work hours must not exceed 80 hours per week, 2) residents may not work more than 24 consecutive hours, 3) there may be exceptions to the 24-hour-shift rule if patient care would be compromised, 4) scheduled rotations must be separated by 8 hours off, and 5) residents must be given one day off per week

In 1987, the Accreditation Council on Graduate Medical Education (ACGME) appointed a task force on resident hours and supervision to review current educational conditions regarding resident supervision and resident work hours. The imposition of such specific work rules had never before been a part of ACGME's role. Recommendations were promulgated in the form of a directive to the individual residency review committees, suggesting that the following policies would help to achieve an appropriate educational environment:

- Residents should be allowed to spend, on average, at least one full day out of seven out of the hospital;
- Residents on average should be assigned on call duty in the hospital no more frequently than every third night; and
- There should be adequate backup if sudden and unexpected patient care needs create resident fatigue sufficient to jeopardize patient care during or following on-call periods.

Review of these recommendations implies that the residency review committees wanted to allow individual programs significant freedom to determine how they would implement the proposed recommendations. The ACGME therefore charged each of the residency review committees to outline specific standards for each specialty, presumably using the limitations set out by the task force on resident hours and supervision as a guide. The ultimate impact of the efforts to reduce resident hours nationally remains uncertain. At present, no clear-cut, exact standards exist for the regulation of resident hours. Within an individual residency program, call schedules still vary among individual hospital rotations.

— TIM'S THOUGHTS —

The key question to be addressed here is the expanded liability for the conduct of fatigued residents. Both the discrepancy in standards across the states and among specialties as well as the possible delay in enforcement or implementation of applicable proposals may leave resident-physicians exposed to liability. An example will highlight this:

A third-year internal medicine resident working in the coronary care unit after being on call for 24 hours is called to place a Swan-Ganz catheter. The staff physician is not available. Several attempts are required. The patient develops a pneumothorax. A chest tube is placed, but an air leak persists. The patient develops an empyema and requires surgical decortication. Postoperatively, the patient dies. There was no monitoring of the Swan-Ganz catheter placement by a senior fellow or staff physician.

Negligence is the failure to possess and exercise the requisite degree of skill and knowledge in caring for a patient. The standard against which the physician's performance is measured is established by expert testimony on the accepted principles of diagnosis, management, or therapy for a given medical condition. The trier of fact decides, as an issue of fact, what the standard of care is in each case, and whether the physician defendant comports with that standard.

Let's limit the discussion to negligence in terms of resident-physician liability. Assuming a hospital has instituted measures to limit resident hours, can the liability be shifted to the resident if he or she knowingly violates the work duration limit, thereby absolving the hospital of liability? The answer is likely no.

First, ACGME's policy to limit resident hours and enforce the policy would be thwarted if the liability were shifted to the resident. Second, the legal doctrine of respondent superior establishes that employers are responsible for the negligent acts of their employees. However, the resident might be found negligent for continuing to function in a sleep-deprived state. Such malpractice claims may continue to follow residents through their attempts to become board certified and obtain licensure. The sobering prospect of bearing liability for mistakes they make when they have exceeded the work time limits should deter residents from ignoring such rules. The personal and professional degradation experienced during malpractice litigation should be another deterrent, even if there is no personal financial responsibility.

The Libby Zion case led to a national crusade to reform the workload and long hours of young doctors. Although the exact facts can be difficult to discern long after the event, reports suggest that Libby had a history of depression and cocaine use and that she was admitted to the New York hospital with fever, chills, and agitation. She may have had a serotonin crisis. Her condition remained undiagnosed, but two young doctors gave her a painkiller, sedative, and restraints—a plan approved on the phone by a senior clinician.

Would a senior physician have been able to put the pieces of the Libby Zion puzzle together? The Libby Zion case focused on residents' sleep deprivation, but missed the elephant in the room: young, inexperienced doctors cannot be expected to make complex diagnoses. That is why they are physicians in training in the first place. Sleep deprivation is one issue, but the larger issue is focused oversight and teaching in the development of young physicians. The take home points for you the resident from this discussion are important. Remember you are a physician in training. You should always seek counsel from senior physicians when facing complex medical problems or when performing high-risk procedures. In my opinion the response that no one is available is never acceptable. Interns and residents must demand help when facing complex, life-threatening clinical scenarios.

— ELIZABETH'S THOUGHTS —

It was during my residency training that the transition to work hour restrictions (80 hours per week averaged over four weeks and no more than 24 hours per call) was put in place. Having experienced both sides of the fence, I understand the pros and cons of restricted and unrestricted work hours. To accommodate for the work-hour restrictions, many residency programs have been forced to adopt a shift-work type of schedule in which one trainee works for a 12-hour shift and then another trainee comes on for the next 12-hour shift. This type of schedule works well with acute care settings such as the Emergency Department because it's a triage-type of service in which the ER physician is expected to appropriately evaluate and treat or triage the patient to another service in a timely fashion.

However, for more prolonged medical requirements such as the inpatient setting, this creates a less-than-ideal situation that results in multiple hand-offs and lack of ownership. When residents were "on call" in the era of unrestricted hours, they were expected to stay overnight; admit the patients; carry through with the workup for their illness, including orderings labs and imaging studies; and follow up on these results and streamline therapies based on these results. They then had to round on their patients in the morning and present them to the attending.

Because the admitting resident had to be there physically to present the patient case and explain the management that ensued based on the speculated diagnosis to the attending, extra effort and caution were taken to thoroughly understand the patient's history, avoid careless mistakes, and appropriately work up and treat the patient. Knowing that you had to answer for your actions made you take ownership of the patients that were under your care.

As an intern, I had to face the expectations of both my upper resident and attending for the care I provided to the patients I was assigned to admit. As an upper resident, I had to face the expectations of my attending while taking responsibility for the actions of my intern when it came to patient care.

When a patient is admitted, everyone on the medical hierarchy was equally responsible for that patient's well-being and management to the level of expertise that is acceptable for their level of training. It was a chance to see your patient's progress from admission to discharge and obtain feedback on the clinical decisions you had made. There was only one hand-off—the one your team made to the oncoming on-call team—and you made this hand-off only after you'd finished rounds with the attending physician and completed all the necessary work needed on your patients.

There was a certain level of pride if your team was known as the responsible team and others did not have to clean up after your mess. There was something to be said for those long call days as well. They helped you bond with the fellow resident or intern who was on with you and a certain sense of comradery formed as you made it through the tiring call together.

TRANSITION TO SHIFT WORK

The transition to shift work transpired during the course of my residency. Instead of an intern and resident working as a team and being on call together, the new team dynamics consisted of one upper-level resident and two interns. During call days, the interns worked in 12-hour shifts—one came in at 7 a.m. and left at 7 p.m. and the overnight one came in at 7 p.m. and left at 7 a.m. The resident worked a 24-hour shift.

As I did wards with this new setup, I noted changes not only with my team, but across the residency in general. The history and physical notes became progressively shorter, especially from the overnight interns who knew they did not have to be there to present their patient's story, or answer questions from the attending the following morning. The morning intern lacked full understanding of the cases of patients who were admitted overnight. Ordering labs or follow-up on the results fell through the cracks as one intern assumed the other would do it.

Some interns rushed to get their work done so as to avoid a "work hour violation," leading to suboptimal communication and care. Interns who had good work ethics and stayed late to care for their patients were reprimanded for violating their work hours. For the interns who were not as dedicated, the new work hour rules served as an excuse for abandoning patient care.

The work-hour restriction stemmed from concerns that inappropriate medical decision were made out of sleep deprivation. During my experience with the new work-hour restrictions, I can't help but question whether having adequate amounts of sleep actually result in better clinical judgment or decisions, especially at the expense of patient ownership. Don't get me wrong, I remember the feeling of exhaustion when a progress note that would typically take me 15 minutes to type up turned into a 60-minute ordeal. However, to me, that was an exercise in being able to recognize my own limitations.

If I had a light call after a few hours of sleep and could think with clarity and knew I could perform a necessary procedure such as a central line in a safe and appropriate manner, I did it. However, if I had busy night without any sleep and was fatigued beyond words, I felt no shame in letting my attending or colleagues know and asking for their help in making medical decisions or doing a procedure. Recognizing your limitations is critical. Oftentimes, because patients and ancillary staff look up to us and we do not want to disappoint, it becomes difficult to say "I don't know" or "I need help." But if a management or procedure is outside your scope of knowledge or capabilities, it is critical to recognize limitations.

PONDERING THE SOLUTION

Are work-hour restrictions the solution? The answer to this question requires deeper investigations as to the logistics and pitfalls of the current healthcare system as a whole, not just the work hours of a sleep-deprived resident. This brings to mind Simpsons' paradox in which a general trend may appear to be the conclusion, but if you break down its individual components, you will find variable results that don't necessarily add up to the big picture.

In this era of readily available tests and algorithms, much of the critical-thinking process is taken out of the equation. Snap judgments and clinical decisions likely are made without much thought. The age-old question of "will this test make a difference in my medical management?" is often thrown out the window in exchange for a "quick rule out" that a CT scan or lab test can provide for us. Why investigate the true underlying etiology of a patient's illness when so many medications are available to cover up whatever superficial problem they're presenting with? With the business aspect of medicine interjecting itself into the academic hospitals, there is an added pressure to perform procedures for revenue with the medico-legal aspect of medicine serving as lighter fluid for this fire of inappropriate testing.

With all these factors in play, it's no wonder that today's trainees become almost conditioned to make brash decisions to get through. Perhaps the answer isn't necessarily a work-hour restriction. Perhaps it's about returning to the foundation set forth by the founders of our current residency program and taking the time to understand quality, not quantity, medicine. Perhaps it means requiring more supervision and involvement from attending physicians. Perhaps it's about applying the principle of essentialism to medicine and trying to eliminate the noise: the mountain of paperwork and documentation physicians and trainees are expected to complete on daily basis.

With the advent of the work-hour restrictions, I went from a system in which I simply worked and took care of patients to a system in which I have to remind myself on a daily or weekly basis to go onto a computer to log my duty hours, lest I face a "professionalism" violation. The bottom line is this: work-hour restrictions alone are probably not going to change the topography of medical care by churning out more responsible and well-trained physicians.

CHAPTER 12

What Risks Do You Face In Your Future?

T he rapid-fire pace of medical practice puts physicians at risk for errors in judgment and performance of procedural skills that could result in allegations of malpractice. This discussion focuses on how to limit the potential for malpractice allegations. The problem, succinctly stated, is that practicing good medicine is not enough to avoid allegation of malpractice.

MALPRACTICE CONSIDERATIONS

First, every human being makes mistakes and physicians are not immune. Medicine has evolved into a complex, multidisciplinary model of practice, with multiple players and levels of care, including nurse practitioners and physician assistants who assume a greater role in the provision of medical care. Risk-adverse physicians must be concerned not only with their own actions and omissions, but also the activity of those ostensibly under their supervision.

Second, the discipline of medicine is bursting at the seams with tough decisions that must be made in seconds. The complexity lies in the fact that physicians must make prompt decisions from imperfect options, and patients, in an emotional and regressed state, must make difficult decisions when confronted with confusing medical terminology regarding unknown diseases. The susceptibility to "Monday morning quarterbacking" is common in the medical community, where there is an exponential growth of review committees in a medical environment tying reimbursement to "quality." When the outcome of a medical judgment/procedure is suboptimal and emotions are running high, second-guessing is rampant, often irrational, and, in a highly competitive medical marketplace, occasionally vindictive.

Third, even when there is no physician error and the decisions are seemingly routine, the practice of standard of care medicine can occasionally have less-than-desired outcomes. There is always a potential for physical injury, pain, emotional distress, and even death. These outcomes are difficult to ignore and surface suspicion of wrongdoing and a desire for retribution. The unique combination of an untoward outcome, a distrustful patient or family, and a persuasive plaintiff attorney creates a recipe for an allegation of malpractice despite the medical practice meeting the standard of care.

RISK MANAGEMENT PRINCIPLES

The astute physician must understand how to develop practice patterns and behaviors that prevent patient frustrations from turning into burdensome litigation. Physicians should understand the principles of risk management discussed in this chapter and develop a coherent plan to implement these principles to minimize the risk of malpractice allegations. Although some of the advice contained herein may seem obvious, many physicians would like to go back in time and apply these basic, but vital principles.

The doctor-patient relationship is crucial in defining the likelihood of a medical malpractice allegation. The importance of a warm, genuinely caring relationship with your patient and the patient's family cannot be overstated. Cultivating such a relationship is an essential skill for all physicians involved in patient care. Genuine care in acting as a fiduciary to the patient will only increase the quality of medical care offered and delivered. The greater the emotional bond between the patient and the physician, the more likely a trusting relationship will evolve and surface all the information needed to allow the physician to identify the correct diagnosis and provide optimal medical care.

Patients sense whether the physician is totally engaged in their medical care. There is empirical evidence that a major determinant in patient satisfaction with the doctor-patient relationship is the patient's perception of the physician's commitment to the communication process. Increasing the emotional connection with the patient enables physicians to practice responsive and paramount medical care, and erects a barrier to an allegation of malpractice in cases of questionable outcomes.

Conversely, if a physician is perceived as arrogant, uninterested, impatient, or blunt with the patient and family, it becomes easy for the patient or patient's family to perceive the physician as callous or reckless. Under these circumstances, any offers of condolence after the fact will fall on deaf ears and will not affect decisions to pursue legal action.

Physicians must develop a content and manner of communication that cultivates a caring relationship. Specifically, physicians must educate patients about the process of care with facilitation of patient/family opinions, checking understanding and encouraging dialogue. Remember, as in all human relationships, honey works better than vinegar.

INFORMED CONSENT

Carefully articulated informed consent that educates the patient about risks and benefits of treatment options, along with documentation, is essential to limiting risk. All informed consent documents should be clearly written and easily understood by the patient and guardian. Physicians must identify that the consent is correctly filled out and reflects a careful and detailed explanation of the medical treatment or procedure with all attendant risks.

In addition to the consent form, it behooves the physician to have a medical record reflecting that the physician informed the patient of all risks and benefits of the treatment and of the patient's understanding and willingness to proceed.

Finally, a physician should prepare an informed consent form that documents a refusal of treatment. In medical malpractice cases, if the consent form does not identify all the risks and alternative approaches to treatment, the physician will have a challenging evidentiary burden proving that the patient was made aware of the risks and alternate approaches to treatment.

DOCUMENTATION

Although often tedious and time-consuming, proper documentation of all aspects of medical care is indispensable. First, it is good medicine and allows serial assessments to be more fruitful. Second, proper documentation allows for more efficient practice because the physician does not need to reinvent the wheel with each patient visit. The ability to recall the details of the last visit suggests to the patient an engaged, caring physician.

Documentation is often the "lifeline" when claims materialize. Memory and evidence are likely to conflict in key respects and credibility of evidence may rest on the accuracy of record documentation. The bottom line in medical malpractice cases is if it is not documented, it did not happen.

THE SECOND OPINION

The judicious, discerning physician who wants to minimize exposure to malpractice claims will graciously accept a patient's desire to seek a second medical opinion. The more grave the prognosis or complex the medical/surgical issues, the more fertile the ground for second guessing physician decisions and actions. It is in precisely such cases that the physician should demonstrate candid commitment to the patient's wellbeing. The physician should encourage and facilitate the second opinion.

The confident, competent physician has nothing to lose and everything to gain by encouraging a second opinion. There is always benefit to additional evaluation of complex problems. The saying, "two minds are better than one" is never so true.

THE STANDARD OF CARE

Physicians are facing increasing pressure to conform their care to insurer or employer guidelines and regiments. It is often a Sisyphean effort to determine whether a particular medical test or procedure is authorized. This can lead to the denial of the most accurate test and can put the physician in the uncomfortable position of falling below the threshold for meeting the standard of care. When such conflicts arise, the physician should pursue all available resources to meet the fiduciary responsibility to the patient and document those efforts, as well as the responses.

Medical informed consent is essential to the physician's ability to diagnose and treat patients effectively, as well as the patient's right to accept or cull the outlined treatment strategy. Medical informed consent should be an exchange of information and ideas that supports the doctor-patient relationship. Physicians should recognize that informed medical consent is an education process and has the potential to develop a doctor-patient coalition to the benefit of the patient and the doctor. When physicians take medical informed consent sincerely, the doctor-patient relationship becomes a true partnership with shared decision-making authority and responsibility for outcomes.

TRANSPARENCY

Physicians with a mindset of complete transparency will develop approaches to patient management that minimize the potential for adverse outcomes. The reporting of medical errors and near misses is an important element in the prevention of future, similar errors, and thus to patient safety. Individual physicians and healthcare institutions should report all medical errors and safety lapses to study the adverse effects and learn preventive measures, and share their findings with other healthcare professionals to eliminate future occurrences. This broad-based sharing would help reveal the root causes of medical errors and allow for the development of methods and guidelines to prevent future physicians from making similar medical errors. Physicians who join the "transparency team" will be less likely to commit medical errors because they will be engaged in the development of protocols, checklists, and strategies to ensure informed consent, comprehensive documentation, crisis-management skills, and knowledge of how to discuss a bad outcome.

CRISIS MANAGEMENT

If and when the course of events in a medical or surgical treatment goes awry, it is imperative that a physician be prepared and equipped to manage the crisis to avoid exacerbating the circumstance and to minimize the potential for harm to the patient. Akin to the captain of a team, the physician must demonstrate leadership by taking charge, assigning priorities, and delegating responsibility. The communication between the health team members must be clear and concise, making certain the messages delivered are received and understood. The essence of teamwork is a must when managing a medical crisis and all involved participants must understand their role and their limitations.

The use of checklists is essential because cognitive skills are less precise in life-and-death circumstances. The development of good crisis management skills should include in-service training and crisis stimulation drills to prepare the staff for unexpected events and outcomes. The time spent drilling these scenarios will result in improved quality, minimization of risk for the patient, and reduced likelihood of liability for the physician

DISCUSSING THE BAD OUTCOME

When Mr. Brown had his mitral valve replaced, the surgery and initial postoperative course were uneventful. A tiny bacterial infection found a home on his prosthetic valve. This might or might not occur as a result of negligence. The operating physician was unaware of this infection, as Mr. Brown had no complaints and was convalescing uneventfully.

Unfortunately, a few weeks after the hospitalization, the bacterial infection embolized to the brain, resulting in a fatal cerebral infarction. The death was totally unexpected and Mr. Brown's wife and family were in shock. They bombard the physician with questions: Why did the bacteria develop in the first place? Why did the embolism cause his death? Was this a preventable situation? The physician was emotionally drained and genuinely shocked at the result.

Many competing interests must be balanced in this delicate situation. The physician must double his efforts to communicate compassionately with the patient and the patient's family when an unfortunate outcome occurs. The words chosen should ideally flow from the relationship that was cultivated before the bad result.

The importance of being caring, sympathetic, and transparent cannot be overstated. Patients and families want to understand what occurred and why. The better their education during the informed consent process, the less likely conflict will surface and the potential for allegations of malpractice.

CHAPTER 13

Doctor—It's Your Own Life

The time to start planning the trajectory of your life is *now*. Consider identifying your plan by sitting down and writing your obituary. What would you want it to say? Start planning your life from the perspective of a family, work-life balance, and personal goals. Identify what is important and eliminate all nonessentials as you plan your life. The plan should have a clear focus and perspective that evolves from a conscious decision about how you will spend your time on this earth. There must be careful consideration of others and oneself. The development of a plan is akin to writing your own life story.

We must create time to escape and explore all the questions and possibilities that make up our life's decisions. This focus must be similar to how our eyes focus: not a fixation on one object, but a constant adjustment and adaptation to the field of vision so we can carefully consider the impact of all possibilities. This is more and more difficult in our over-stimulated world.

The paradox is that the faster and busier things become, the more important it is that we take time to build time into our day for focused thinking. The noisier things become the more important it is that we build in reflection time so we can identify the signals amongst the noise of daily life. This thinking space allows us to reflect on the big picture: where we are and where we are going with family, work, and personal choices. In the chaos of the modern world and work place with many demands pulling us in multiple directions, it is more important than ever to resist distraction and remain focused on the essentials of our life.

It is imperative that you protect your assets such as your health and emotional tranquility. Sleep is a priority; it promotes creativity and allows for the highest level of mental and physical function. Learn to be selective, explicit, and systematic in how you spend your time. Eliminate all things that are not essential to you. Learning to say *no* is critical to high performance.

Identify where you can maximize your use of time and energy—this allows you to live with your intent. Setting boundaries allows you to limit the noise of others and have the time to pursue your dreams. Remove all obstacles that interfere with your global plan for your family, your friends, and your work. Focus on the present, tuning into what is important and enjoying the moment. This is your life and it is up to you to do it your way. Invest in your future.

TIM AND ELIZABETH'S UNIFYING CONCEPTS

Action Steps:

- Become an essentialist
- Learn the necessary intelligences
- Understand the importance of mental and physical health
- Put your family first
- Make sure you have a life-long learning curve
- Be a fiduciary—always put patients first
- Respect and develop the healthcare team
- Understand the concepts where law and medicine intersect
- Understand the importance of preventive healthcare
- Give back to the community
- Make your defining feature generativity—the concern for establishing and guiding the next generation

Part Four

The Present State
and the Future
of Healthcare

CHAPTER 14

The Changing Face of Healthcare

Immortalized in books and perpetuated through the media, doctoring is often portrayed as a glorifying profession of healing patients, achieving academic excellence, and epitomizing the definition of humanity.

Yet for those living and practicing the life of a physician, it's a different story. Many are burned out, dissatisfied, and often wondering if they made the right decision going into this profession. The sense of satisfaction derived from the improvement of a patient's illness through your management is often fleeting, as it is replaced by the constraint and stresses of administrative pressures to see more patients, do more tests, and complete endless amounts of documentation for "medical-legal" and "quality of care" purposes.

The doctor-patient relationship has shifted, and many physicians feel helpless at the mercy of their patients and corporate medicine. Physician blogs are filled with stories about frustrating experiences within the medical field. Physicians go into this profession thinking it would be an opportunity to learn about human diseases, take care of patients and make them better, and go home at the end of the day with a certain sense of purpose in life. Instead, many feel like they know less and less about their patients as they drown in more and more electronic "paperwork." Patients don't seem to be satisfied with their care and at the end of the day, many physicians go home feeling dejected and tired rather satisfied with having served some type of purpose.

WHAT HAS HAPPENED?

To understand the transformation to the current day healthcare landscape, we need to look at the processes involved in the evolution of the healthcare system. Kenneth H. Ludmerer, in *Let Me Heal,* provides great insight into this question by exploring the history of medical care and the development of training programs for doctors that led to the current infrastructure for residency training. The book also reflects the overall changes and challenges of the entire healthcare system as a whole.

Prior to the mid-19th century, medical training and education came in the form of an apprenticeship in in which "house officers," what medical apprentices were called, would often observe and follow the orders of a seasoned physician without assuming much of the clinical responsibilities themselves. There was no set curriculum and education was variable. Many house officers felt resentment as their quest for education and autonomy was met by consternation and more labor from their attending. The balance of their educational needs versus their institution's objective for cheap labor was a major point of contention.

This changed in the last part of the 19th century with the advent of medical school. The impetus for scholarly aspirations and scientific exploration came from Europe. American physicians who had the opportunity to study abroad brought back inspirations from Europe where there were established systems of rigorous medical training and academic research to support their clinical practices.

From this idea, Johns Hopkins, through the planning of William Osler, William Halstead, Howard Kelly, and Henry Hurd, created the first graduate medical program in 1889. It was the Renaissance of medical training. Candidates were accepted to the program only if they showed not only academic excellence but scientific aptitude—meaning that intelligence and good grades alone would not have sufficed. They had to show an ability to expand their thinking outside of what was conventional and possess a sense of investigation.

Once accepted, house officers were expected to live in the hospital during the term of their training. This meant they spent their days in the hospital not only working, caring for patients, and studying, but also eating, sleeping, and developing friendships there. The residents were more than content to do this, with their disposition described as "monks in a happy monastery."

WHY WAS IT LIKE THIS?

It was a different time, situation, and mindset. Since it was such a privilege to be accepted, many saw this as a "calling" rather than as a career or apprenticeship. It was a life of devotion to a cause. Additionally, the training environment is one that's especially different from today. It was an "Oslerian" time when all the faculty and staff were deeply caring and invested in their house officers. In turn, the house officers felt a deep-seated commitment to not only their patients but the attending physicians whose tutelage they were under.

This is the real-life example of "mirror cells" as discussed in Chapter 2 in which the positivity of one entity is reflected in another. The house officers were more than eager to put in the hours and work because the attending physicians invested the same in teaching and promoting the growth of their pupils.

With time, the medical system rapidly grew and with this expansion came a sense of depersonalization as academic health centers hired more faculties and compartmentalized into "specialized" departments to accommodate the larger volumes of patients. The increased number of patients came as a response to the enactment of Medicare and Medicaid.

The exchange rate for a prosperous academic hospital center came at the cost of dissipated genteel collegiality and dilution of teachings and education to the residents. Trainees were working the arduous hours of their predecessors of the Oslerian time, but felt their labors were not rewarded with the learning they had hoped to receive in return.

Today, the patient load significantly increased as the turnover continues to rise. Length of hospitalization has significantly decreased—not necessarily due to better care, but increased pressure from hospital administration to be profitable. Residents now see more patients and in exchange have less time to explore their history and physical exam findings, and ponder on the differentials. Instead, there is a rush to make expedited medical decisions, complete paperwork to fulfill quality of care measures, and other social issues that eluded residency of Osler's time.

Residents spend countless hours working, but are not necessarily invested in the care of patients, or exploring their illnesses or treatment. Instead, much of time is spent completing the necessary tasks to grease the wheels of the hospital factory. Likewise, many attending physicians are faced with the same administrative pressures to meet certain quotas of productivity that consume much of their time. Consequently, some are burned out and find it difficult to meet expectations of their bosses while allotting the time needed to teach their trainees.

It is a trickle-down effect that starts with the hospital corporate "leaders" who make policies and decisions as to what is expected of their physician employees. Those specializing in business rather than patient care ("managerialists)—those who are out of touch with clinical medicine are making many of these decisions and policies. These policies and quotas are then forced upon the physicians, with some struggling to balance the humanistic aspect of patient care and doctoring with corporate expectations of perceived productivity.

The burden of responsibility then trickles down to trainees, as ancillary duties are then passed on to them and the time for educating them is sacrificed in order for attending physicians to meet their own objectives to satisfy their bosses. To compound this deteriorating situation, to reduce budgeting costs, many hospitals may choose to not hire additional staffing support in the form of social workers, case managers, nurses, nurse practitioners, and physician assistants, since the salary of some of these personnel is more than what is paid to a resident. Again, the residents are left to absorb the lack of staffing as their job expectations increase to other ancillary duties of filling out the necessary paperwork for not only the patient's medical issues (i.e., prescriptions, admission/discharge orders) but also social issues (i.e., placement for skilled facility, handicap/disability paperwork).

So despite advances in the medical education system over the years that was so carefully planned by our medical forefathers, we find ourselves in the same conflict that plagued those before the 19th century—the educational and personal needs of the residents and physicians versus the corporate goals of the institution. A historical view reveals we've made a full-circle, but not in a good way.

WHAT WENT WRONG?

Many factors contributed to the deterioration of the chaotic healthcare system that we currently have. Perhaps a better analysis of these factors can help provide an understanding as to what is and what must be done to improve the future of healthcare.

DEPERSONALIZATION

"How can we care for our patients, if nobody cares for us?"—Chuck, *House of God*, Samuel Shem.

The resounding message in what Chuck says is underscored in *Let Me Heal*. It essentially goes back to the golden rule of "Treat others as you would want to be treated yourself." If someone cares for you, in turn, you will care for them. It's the paradigm that underlies the fundamental relationships of human beings and the theories behind human interactions, including that of mirror cells or positive reinforcement.

Think back to Oslerian days when residents were expected to live in the hospital and work copious amounts of hours. They didn't mind because they had attending physicians and mentors who deeply cared for their education and success in advancing up the medical ladder. Contrast it with today's medical training, and there's a certain sense of depersonalization between trainees and their attendings. Accordingly, attendings have the same sense of disconnect with their superiors and hospital administrators. Often this stems from being devalued as physicians. They feel "dispensable" if they do not need the requisite productivity quota.

Most people respond to feeling devalued, or dispensable, by leaving that job, or staying at the job, but performing at the level to just keep their job, but not beyond. This does not imply any physician tries to work in a subpar fashion; however, with the demanding environment of healthcare involving large volumes of patients, mountains of paperwork, and expectations of the hospitals, many physicians feel like they're barely keeping their heads above water. As much as we all want to be better human beings and altruistic, it takes a very special being to not be overwhelmed in the current environment of "healthcare." It becomes almost ironic that a system meant to care for the health and well-being of patients has neglected the well-being of its own employees who makes up a critical component of its infrastructure.

DOCTOR-PATIENT RELATIONSHIP

The doctor-patient relationship is a complex entity that in itself has been discussed extensively in literature and on social media. To better understand this dynamic relationship, let's look at what it was and what it is now.

In the early days of medicine, the doctor-patient relationship was purely a paternalistic one that involved the physician deciding what was best for the patient, and the patient agreeing without much questions or resistance. It was the natural order of things then, especially in an era where medical knowledge was limited only to those privileged enough to obtain training in it. Patients conscientiously accepted their diagnosis and underwent treatment as instructed by their physicians. In turn, many physicians of the time understood their profession to be more of "calling" and their treatment of patients as a sacred covenant.

With advances in technology and the introduction of the World Wide Web, patients now have more access to information on their health, symptoms, and illnesses. Armed with information they can now easily obtain from the Internet, patients have become autonomous in their own healthcare. This caused a shift in the traditional paternalistic doctor-patient relationship, as patients started to challenge the idea that physicians always know what is best.

The doctor-patient relationship has significantly changed over the years, but not necessarily in a positive direction. Like a disintegrating marriage, the relationship is fraught with mistrust, disenchantment, and an overall lack of empathy from both sides. Despite the common goal and desire to make the relationship work harmoniously, often differences or changes in core values as well as extraneous environmental factors such as finances divide both parties.

However, unlike a marriage, physicians and patients cannot divorce themselves from the other entity and just walk away. As a patient, you may have the option to leave a physician that you don't like, but you cannot escape the healthcare system as whole if you expect to have some type of illness in the future that will require medical attention. As a physician, you cannot ignore your patients' discontentment because their well-being is the sole basis for your profession.

Ask patients what is the most important thing they want from their doctors and the majority will answer, *"I want to feel like my doctor really cares about me."* Ask physicians what they want from their patients, and the majority will answer, *"I wish my patients would understand I'm trying my best to care for them."*

There is similarity in the desires of both entities to find some connection with each other. The intent is good, but, that is where the common ground ends between patients and doctors and the disconnect starts. Perhaps in order to remedy the issues that plague this relationship, we need to actually look at the doctor-patient interaction as an actual relationship. In Gary Chapman's, *The 5 Love Languages*, he discusses how two people can have the same objective to make a relationship work, but if they don't speak in a language that appeals to the other person, much of the original intent of the message, no matter how well meaning, will be lost. To deal with this, we need to understand what is meaningful to the other party.

What makes patients feel like their doctors care for them? Many say they want a doctor who takes the time to talk and listen. Empathy and understanding go a long way. Picking on the non-verbal cues as to what's bothering them is perhaps more valuable than prescribing that magic pill that will fix their cholesterol numbers. The psychological well-being is just as important, if not more important than the physical well-being, and sometimes doing nothing goes a longer way than doing everything.

What makes physicians feel good about their profession? Their patients' happiness and health are the positive reinforcement many physicians need to regain meaning.

With the increased patient volume and corporate takeover of medicine, physicians are expected to see an exorbitant number of patients. Because they are now seeing more patients in the same allotted time (after all there are still only 24 hours in a day), physicians must now spend less time with each of their patients to make time for the next.

With less time to spend understanding and exploring patient's ailments, many physicians order multiple tests to "rule out" possible diagnoses or refer their patient to specialists, thereby driving up the costs of healthcare. Specialists, due to their own increasing patient load and just by the very nature of their position in the medical hierarchy, will often focus on only one problem while ignoring the overall clinical picture. In the end, patients end up with expensive medical bills and a list of diagnoses they don't have and no actual answer of what is really going with them. Anyone in this situation would be dissatisfied.

Let's say a patient presents to the emergency department (ED) with complaints of lightheadedness and dizziness. The hospitalist is called for admission and evaluation of the patient. The tired and time-constrained hospitalist who has already seen more than 20 patients that day goes to see this patient in the ED and quickly gets a history and does a physical examination. Based on the patient's complaints of dizziness, near syncope (almost passing out), and increased fatigue an electrocardiogram (ECG) showing a slowed heart rate (bradycardia) and atrioventricular block (AVB), the hospitalist consults the cardiologist. Also, because the patient had complained of some numbness, tingling, and weakness in extremities, the neurologist is also consulted for good measure.

After a non-contrast head CT, MRI, and carotid Doppler's, the neurologist announces that the patient likely does not have a stroke. The cardiologist, focusing on the symptoms of dizziness and nearly passing out with the bradycardia on ECG and telemetry, recommends a pacemaker. Several days later, the patient is discharged with a newly placed pacemaker and feeling better. However, as days go by his joints hurt and the fatigue persists along with intermittent numbness. If the patient is lucky, the next physician who sees him may have the time or astuteness to get a better history from him, put the pieces of puzzle together, and obtain a Lyme antibody test and start antibiotics. If he's not, then the cycle of additional tests and specialists will continue. Perhaps a rheumatologist may be involved this time around.

These situations spark the mistrust patients have towards their physicians. From this mistrust stems questions about a physician's management and from this comes the basis of medical litigation. In response, physicians increase their practice of "defensive medicine" in which they implement unnecessary testing or consultations in order to "not miss anything" should they be challenged in the court of law. In practicing "defensive medicine," physicians manifest their mistrust of patients, the healthcare system, and legal system. The vicious cycle of skepticism and cynicism between patients and doctors is self-perpetuating.

BEING ACCOUNTABLE

How do we break this vicious cycle? Like a marriage, perhaps the answer lies in both parties taking accountability and owning up to their responsibilities to each other.

THE PHYSICIAN

In the current healthcare system, a physician's competency and account-ability is scrutinized from all aspects with various "tools" to assess the quality of that physician. The tools used to assess physicians' academic competency include board exams and continuing medical education (CME) credits. Traditionally, in order to be certified, physicians had to not only have completed medical school and residency, but also pass all the requisite board exams before earning the title of "board certified" for their chosen specialty. Now, to maintain their board-certified status, physicians must retake and pass recertification board exams every 6 to 10 years based on their specialty.

During the years between their board exams, physicians must meet a pre-requisite number of hours benchmarked for CME annually. This system has been further complicated by the introduction of the maintenance of certification (MOC) requirements set out by the medical boards that govern practicing physicians, both medical and surgical. The MOC pro-gram requires that physicians complete the required tests and hours for continuing medical education, but also pay a fee (either a one-time pay-ment to cover for 10 years or annual payments) for the board to "publicly acknowledge" that the physician was certified. Significant controversy arose over these new requirements as physicians felt they were being exploited financially. Additionally, the requirements represented a growing amount of "paperwork" and documentation that physicians already felt inundated by their own workplace.

From a productivity standpoint, physicians are monitored through a "pay per performance" of relative value unit (RVU) point system that attempts to take into account the number of patients, the complexity of their medi-cal problems, and the tests and procedures that are performed on them. Reimbursement for services rendered is commensurate to the number of RVUs accumulated or reported.

The shortcoming of this system lies in the fact that it rewards physicians who perform more tests and procedures on patients without a fail-proof system to assess whether the tests and procedures were appropriate for the situation. By its inherent point system, RVUs promote the practice of unnecessary testing and procedures that are low yield to a patient's healthcare and well-being, thereby perpetuating the vicious cycle of mistrust previously discussed.

To limit fraudulent claims, Medicare closely monitors the trends of physician reporting for their RVUs and required linkage of procedure and tests to appropriate diagnoses. However, this is only a blanket attempt at controlling the wildfire of commercialism that has engulfed the healthcare system.

Another manner of evaluating the performance of doctors comes in the form of "physician report cards" which are released to the public to provide information on the quality of the physician based on hospital metrics and consumer/patient feedback. Superficially, this initiative seems like a great idea to not only provide the public information about the physicians they may be seeing, it also serves as a benchmark to incentivize practitioners to improve themselves and their report card grades. This appeals to those who go into the medical profession and want to achieve their absolute best. Many physicians have professional pride and do what they can to improve their report card grade even at the cost of financial reimbursement. Sounds like a win-win situation all around, right?

Let's take a closer look at what doctors can do to improve their grades. One of the metrics many hospitals look at and can objectively report are mortality rates associated with a particular physician. This is especially important in surgical and procedural specialties in which a more direct correlation can be extrapolated to cause (e.g., surgery resulting in complication) and effect (i.e. death). So let's take a look at the report card of internal medicine physicians or surgeons who are willing to take care of the sickest patients. Their report cards will naturally have a higher mortality rate and hence lower score. Does this truly reflect their humanistic quality as doctors who care for the sickest of us? No, instead it serves as a detriment to them. They can easily remedy this and improve their score by simply refusing to take on the cases of sick patients. But then what happens to these very sick patients? They are left to find a physician who's willing to take on the "liability" of having a bad report card score in favor of appropriate care.

Another metric of physician performance is patient satisfaction. For some patients, being satisfied might come from feeling like their doctor listened to them. For some, satisfaction may come from a short wait time for their appointment. For others, satisfaction may come from their doctors giving them what they're requesting.

Physicians regularly find themselves making medical decisions that their patients disagree with, or are displeased by. A common example is pre-scribing pain medications. Many patients come into their physician's office requesting pain pills and they do so without realizing the truly addictive nature of these medications as they build up tolerance with increasing strength. A physician's ability to be firm and say *no* may be the only safe-guard from dangerous adverse reactions, including death for some of these patients. However, the patients who are told *no* are not happy. In turn, they report their dissatisfaction with the care they received from that physician. So in the end, report cards are not always a true reflection of quality care. They provide a crude approximation of physician quality and performance, but their interpretation must be made with an open mindset of the complex issues that underlie medical care.

THE PATIENT

Despite all the measures of quality of care and performance a physician must achieve, there is not much in way of a "report card" for patients. Why do we need a "report card" for patients? Because if physicians should be held accountable for their role in a relationship, so should the other par-ticipating party.

An epidemic problem that physicians face when it comes to patient care is adherence—whether it's adherence to a healthier lifestyle, or to prescribed medications. Research demonstrates that non-adherence to long-term medications accounts for an estimated preventable cost of more than $300 billion annually. Much of this comes in the form of re-hospitalizations for chronic medical problems, as well as complications that occur as a result of poorly controlled chronic illnesses, such as heart failure, hypertension and diabetes.

Classic examples of this include patients with known heart failure and reduced left ventricular systolic function who continue to consume salty foods, or forget to take their medications, and must be admitted for their acute decompensated heart failure, or those with chronic obstructive pulmonary disease who continue to smoke cigarettes and come in for exacerbations that require nebulized breathing treatments, steroids, and antibiotics.

Yet there is not a standardization of reporting for patients to demonstrate that they are doing their part in preventing the escalation of the adverse consequences of their illness.

REDEFINING THE DOCTOR-PATIENT RELATIONSHIP

The paternalistic manner of medicine in which doctors dictate the care of patients creates an imbalanced relationship where patients feel helpless and at the mercy of the often-biased decision-making process of their physicians. The decision-making process needs to be a joint venture of both physicians and patients.

With the wealth of literature on health and illnesses readily available to the public, patients are more knowledgeable than ever about the normal physiology and pathophysiology of their bodies. Eric Topol, in his forward thinking book *The Patient Will See You Now*, discusses the use of the most popular technology into the healthcare system: smartphones and apps. He advocates that patients take charge of their own healthcare through the easily accessible digital world of applications and medical resources. He encourages "democratization" of medical knowledge through large networks to allow information sharing and discussion to dissipate overall medical costs. He predicts the future landscape of healthcare to be dictated by patients via mobile devices that would allow patients access to their medical records and easily obtainable labs.

In the end, the patient-doctor interaction is still a relationship. As is the natural behavior of relationships, the preservation of balance of power is crucial to reinforce positivity. An imbalance can only be sustained for a certain period time before resistance against it develops.

We need to acknowledge the strengths of both physicians and patients and utilize them to their fullest potential. The strength of patients is that they know their bodies better than any physician will during a 30 minute or even hour visitation. Patients should take the time to understand their symptoms and what it might mean in the context of their own body. They should be their own medical record keeper, gather readily available digital literature and adopt a more active role in their own healthcare. Physicians should appreciate this aspect of their patients, take the time to listen to the information they're presenting, accept their challenges with open mind, and whole-heartedly encourage their active participation in the joint decision-making process.

The strength of the physician is sheer experience. After years of education, training, and practice, physicians have witnessed firsthand diseases in patients and their natural progression. It is this experience that allows physicians to appreciate the multifaceted nature of diseases.

As many physicians will attest to, reading about diseases and their clinical presentation and treatment is completely different than dealing with them in real time. The old axiom of diseases "not following the book" rings true in the majority of patient cases and it's usually a more seasoned physician who will pick up on the nuances to make the correct diagnosis.

Although digital and biotechnological advances may enhance our ability to detect diseases, or monitor for them, it cannot completely replace the complex thought processes and mental associations that can only come from human thought and experiences.

Though it will not be an easy task, it is a necessary endeavor for both physicians and patients to work together and change their way of thinking and actions in order to improve the current state of our disintegrating healthcare system.

CHAPTER 15

The Physician's Role in Changing Health Behaviors

"Everything should be made as simple as possible, but not simpler."

—Albert Einstein

With advances in biotechnology, the average life expectancy is significantly longer today than in the past. As practicing cardiologists, we observe firsthand that even though there are artificial means to prolong our patients' lives, they are still prematurely aging at an alarming rate. Many are sedentary, overweight, deconditioned, and apathetic. Consequently, they experience heart attacks, strokes, musculoskeletal injuries, cancers, and premature death.

The soaring healthcare costs and epidemics of obesity, heart diseases, and cancer are lifestyle-related. Approximately 70% of disease and death is related to lifestyle choices, including heart disease, strokes, diabetes, obesity, and musculoskeletal maladies. We could eliminate more than 50% of these illnesses if we had the constitutional fabric to make healthy behavioral choices. Idleness and fast food are killing us.

As physicians, we do what we are trained to do very well—we treat disease. Our training exposes us to every complex disease known to humankind and we learn the methods to control or cure these diseases. However, for a large majority of these patients, their problems are the result of lifestyle choices. Patients would rather take pills or insulin shots to control their diabetes than make the necessary dietary and lifestyle modifications to consume more nutrient-dense foods, increase exercise, and lose weight. Lack of discipline to make the quintessential lifestyle changes is a significant problem because it leads to epidemics of obesity and coronary artery disease.

Most of modern medicine is transactional. You experience a heart attack and undergo stenting or bypass surgery with a short period for recovery and everyone goes their own way. This transactional approach to medicine is failing patients. The winners are corporate medicine and the losers are patients. The answer was simple: we need to identify how to seek health.

The merit of an idea does not predict its adoption. The greatest barrier to any change lies in the continued acceptance of poorly thought-through decisions. Unhealthy "normative behavior" such as eating at fast food restaurants is sustained by a culture that is running on a hedonic treadmill at a rapid pace toward the unsatisfactory solutions of stents and coronary artery bypass surgery. Change will languish until the community can take direct action to embrace a new paradigm based on knowledge.

The first step is recognition with open discourse. We must break the code of silence that sustains the status quo of fast food joints and couch surfing. We must spread the word. Members of every community must share their insights and views openly. We must jump off the hedonic treadmill now.

The second step in creating this new healthy norm is to make *everyone accountable* by publically encouraging healthy behavior and openly confronting the unhealthy behavior. The strength of the new norm depends on the consistency with which the community and community leaders are willing to speak up, act together, and lead through example. The entire village must embrace a whole new culture of healthy behavior. The challenge to change must be met by all of us together.

EVERY PATIENT AN ATHLETE

Why identify every patient an athlete? Athletes are perceived to be the healthiest members of our society. Prototypically, athletes have unique mental and physical characteristics that allow them to achieve peak performance. The truth is every single patient has an inner child waiting to become an athlete. Healthcare professionals must teach and mentor their patients in healthy eating habits and training routines necessary to become a heart healthy "athlete."

First we must explore the unique characteristics of athletes. Athletes have a burning desire to be the best. They possess a deep commitment to always improving, taking their performance to the next level. The only standard for an athlete is excellence. They perceive no obstacles, only challenges to overcome. Failure is not an option. Taking on risks and pushing beyond their comfort zone is part of the championship mind. Athletes eat healthy foods and train to high levels to obtain peak mental, physical, and emotional function and peak performance in their sport. Clearly, our patients need these characteristics as they pursue healthy eating and regular exercise to seek optimal health.

For your patients desiring optimum health, physical energy is the fuel that drives alertness, vitality, and an ability to manage emotions, sustain concentration, think creatively, and maintain a mindset through superior brain executive function to obtain optimum health. The physical energy galvanizes the mental energy necessary to maintain the willpower needed to exercise and eat healthy on a sustained basis. The physical and mental energy are synergistic, taking athletes to optimum performance. Let's explore how proper eating and exercise can help our patients.

A critical source of physical energy comes from the types of food we eat. Balanced, healthy eating allows us to function effectively mentally and physically. Foods high in sugars and simple carbohydrates are less energy-rich than proteins and complex carbohydrates. It is important to eat low glycemic foods. The glycemic index measures the rate with which the sugars from specific foods are released into the bloodstream. A slow release is desired to provide a constant source of energy for the body.

The lowest glycemic foods that provide the highest and longest source of energy include whole grains, protein-rich foods, and low glycemic fruits such as pears, grapefruit, and apples. High glycemic foods such as muffins, bagels, and sugary cereals create a spike in energy for a short period of time, but ultimately prompt a blood sugar crash and promote inflamma-tion. A traditional breakfast of an unbuttered bagel and a glass of orange juice, which is often viewed as "healthy," is high on the glycemic index and results in an energy debt and inflammation.

How often we eat influences our capacity to stay fully engaged physically, mentally, and emotionally, and to attain and sustain high performance activities. Eating six low-calorie, highly nutritious, low glycemic meals per day ensures a steady supply of energy. Waiting six to eight hours between meals leaves an individual in a state of fuel deficit and promotes suboptimal mental and physical performance. Sustaining mental and physical energy depends on eating as frequently as you need to fuel the next three hours.

Portion control is critical in managing weight and regulating energy levels for optimum mental and physical performance. Snacks between meals should focus on low glycemic foods such as nuts, apples, and protein bars. The goal is to have a brain satiety center that is never hungry, or full.

Water is an excellent source of energy and provides health and longevity benefits. Thirst is a suboptimal barometer of hydration. By the time we are thirsty, we are dehydrated. Dehydrate a muscle 3%, and it will lose 10% of its strength and 8% of its speed and efficiency of function at the cellular level. Dehydration impairs concentration and mental acuity. Drinking 64 ounces of water every day enhances mental and physical performance and ultimately health.

What about regular exercise? Exercise interval training has enormous physical, mental, and emotional benefits. The theory behind interval training is to engage in short to moderate periods of intense, sustained exercise alternating with short periods of reduced level of exercise intensity. This interval training promotes alternating heart rate levels and promotes efficient recovery of aerobic metabolism. Both cardiovascular aerobic training and resistance strength training have powerful benefits on health, energy levels, and mental and physical performance. Interval training allows us to build more energy capacity and tolerate more stress. Rhythmicity trains the human body to recover more efficiently.

Strength training is as important as cardiovascular training because loss of muscle mass and loss of physical strength is connected to aging and reduced energy capacity. We believe cardiovascular and strength training are mandatory and should be performed every other day, and that exercise training should occur six days per week. This exercise training becomes a self-fulfilling activity, prompting positive emotions that result in peak mental and physical performance.

It is well documented in the medical literature that we derive physical and mental benefit from moderate exercise. This fact in isolation mandates that we as healthcare professionals must educate and mentor our patients to become heart-healthy athletes. We must also asses the risk of exercise for our patients before implementing an exercise regimen. The screening requires an in-depth understanding of the potential issues that could result in adverse health outcomes from exercising. To date, screening markers have marginal clinical benefit in determining risk. Most markers are correlated with traditional risk factors and therefore do not have high independent odds ratios (relative risk).

A screening test should not be considered a diagnostic test, but a triage and reclassification test. Triage is a test used before an existing diagnostic test is preformed, and only patients with a particular result on the triage test continue down the diagnostic pathway. A triage-screening test does not aim to improve the accuracy of the diagnostic test; it reduces the need for additional testing that may be expensive and invasive.

Each patient must be evaluated with a comprehensive personal and family history as well as a complete physical examination that allows synthesis of this information to determine risk and what further testing is necessary. The personalized assessment must assess the risk for coronary artery disease and structural heart disease. Coronary artery disease is the number one cause of death in men and women in our society.

For the general adult population, the American Heart Association Guidelines for adults recommend risk assessment beginning at age 40 and repeated every 5 years, or sooner if there is any emerging risk concern. However, in older competitive athletes (>35 years old) recurring assessment may be more important.

For young athletes, recommendations include cardiovascular (CV) screening every two years with an abbreviated examination in intervening years. Overall the detection of pre-emergent CV disease has become a polarized public health debate, triggering a large and growing body of literature, including clinical studies, editorials, opinion pieces, proclamations, and reviews on both sides of the question.

Although echocardiography is the most robust noninvasive cardiovascular exam and multi-feature biomarker, it is perfunctorily excluded or considered second tier because of inaccessibility, cost, and inter-observer variability. However, echocardiography is recognized as the single most useful diagnostic test in the evaluation of patients with heart failure. This designation of "most useful test" would also apply to more than 90% of all remaining conditions associated with sudden death in athletes.

Echo/Doppler is a readily accessible, reproducible pathophysiologic test, and universal biomarker, which complements its role as a first order CV anatomic and hemodynamic tool. The cardiovascular community has consistently acknowledged that echocardiography has the validated potential to be the best all round screening test if the three fundamental impediments of access, cost, and inter-observer variability were definitively resolved.

We believe Doppler-echocardiography is the most useful test to safely, routinely, and economically quantify diastolic and systolic cardiac function. Echocardiography can detect the common etiologies associated with adverse outcomes with strenuous exercise such as hypertensive heart disease, cardiomyopathies, ischemic heart disease (stress echocardiography), and pulmonary hypertension, coarctation of the aorta, valvular heart disease, anomalous coronary arteries, aortic aneurysm, and congenital heart disease. The testing that depicts pre-clinical disease is diastolic function. Primary diastolic dysfunction occurs early in the emergence of hypertensive heart disease, cardiomyopathies, and ischemic heart disease.

MEETING THE CHALLENGE

The challenge for us as healthcare professionals is huge. The merit of an idea does not predict its adoption. The greatest barrier to any change lies in the continued acceptance of poorly thought-through decisions. Unhealthy "normative behaviors" are sustained by a culture that is running on a hedonic treadmill at a rapid pace toward stents and surgery. Unfortunately stents and surgery generate large sums of money for the corporate suites. Change will continue to languish until the community of healthcare professionals can take direct action to embrace a new paradigm based upon the well-being of our patients.

It is obvious that current behaviors resulting in coronary, metabolic, and obesity epidemics carry an enormous physical, emotional, and financial cost to the human population. Despite this travesty, we persist in activities that not only sustain, but also increase the unhealthy norms. A conspiracy of silence persists as we continue to suffer from these preventable diseases and medical corporations' profits skyrocket.

The first step toward change is open debate and discourse. Our journey together in this book is a healthy step toward change. The next step is for you, the reader, to spread the word to your patients and your communities. Members of your communities must share their insights and views without falling victim to the concerns of public ridicule for stepping outside the ingrained human behaviors and present-day medical paradigms. The message in our communities must be loud and clear—prevention is the best medicine.

The second step in creating a new norm of health is to make everyone accountable by publically encouraging the behaviors we have discussed and openly confronting the sedentary and gluttony behaviors that result in serious, life-threatening diseases. The strength of the new norm depends on the consistency of us spreading the messages in our schools, churches, and medical institutions. We must speak up and act together.

Old norms of gluttony and sedentary behavior will fade fast when the impact of unhealthy behaviors is emphasized in the bright light of public discourse. We implore all healthcare professionals to become leaders in the movement to prevention and health. Providing a portal of information on the Internet to change the healthcare epidemics of obesity and coronary disease will be our gold medal.

Part Five

The Medical Legal System

This section should be read for general knowledge and used as a resource when specific issues arise in daily practice. The purpose of the section is to give a broad and general overview of the law and how it impacts medical practitioners. This virtual tour of the legal system will hopefully help prevent the real-life crisis of intersecting with the legal system.

CHAPTER 16

The Anatomy of a Lawsuit

E very medical practitioner should read this chapter, which takes you through a lawsuit process. The journey through this lawsuit will affect how you practice medicine. It also will give you a new respect for the importance of meeting the standard of care on every patient you encounter in medical practice.

You are a family medicine doctor covering the emergency room. A 49-year-old male arrives at the ER with chest pain. He has no risk factors for coronary artery disease. The nurse relays to you that the vital signs are normal. Blood pressure is 140/85 mm Hg and the heart rate is regular at a rate of 80 bpm.

You interview the patient, identifying he has 3/10 mid sternal chest pain waxing and waning for last 24 hours. You identify no precipitating or alleviating factors to explain the chest pain. The patient appears tense. He denies any significant emotional stress. The cardiopulmonary physical examination is normal. The electrocardiogram (ECG) is normal, as is the chest X-ray. The blood tests, including a troponin level, are normal. The patient states the pain has resolved and he believes it is anxiety related. He wants to be discharged.

You decide the patient is low risk based upon symptoms, physical examination, ECG, and blood tests. You discharge the patient from the emergency room and recommend follow up with his family physician. The next day you learn the patient died of an apparent heart attack.

THE LAW SUIT IS FILED: NOW WHAT?

While the typical response is gloom and despair, and an over-abundance of self-pity, you must reset your thinking and see the seeds of future success in the chaos of alleged negligence.

Litigation is a physician's nightmare—disruptive to a physician's personal and professional life. Physicians feel personally and professionally attacked. Even if a physician prevails at trial, the victory is lost in the devastating emotional cost of alleged liability and ultimate victory can feel like defeat.

No amount of advance knowledge or preparation can alleviate the anxiety and emotional toll of the litigation process; however, knowing the nuisances of the litigation process helps a physician endure and navigate the process.

THE LAWSUIT PROCESS

The Beginning

Claims of negligence are frequently resolved by the insurance carrier without a lawsuit ever being filed. These claims are typically clear-cut examples where the standard of care was breached. When it is unclear whether there was a violation of the standard of care, the litigation process often moves forward. The query surfaced by the allegation of negligence often involves determining who bears responsibility for the alleged negligence. Alternatively, the claimant and insurance companies, and/or physicians cannot agree on the valuation of the claim.

When a patient, or the family of a deceased patient, has determined that the physician's malpractice carrier will not resolve a claim for medical malpractice, the patient or the administrator/executer of the estate will initiate formal legal action by filing a complaint. The patient or executor, known as the plaintiff, will have an attorney file in a state court a complaint describing the factual and legal basis for the lawsuit. There are specific time limitations by which a lawsuit must be filed. A physician should never consider a potential claim "dead" until advised by the insurer, or his or her attorney, that the applicable time to file a lawsuit has expired.

An action against a physician does not begin until the complaint is filed with the court and officially served upon the physician. The proper means of service of a complaint is governed by each state's law and includes being served personally, or by registered, or certified mail. The timing and manner of service is important, as errors in the process of serving the complaint can result in the lawsuit being dismissed (see below). When a physician receives a complaint alleging malpractice, or a letter, or other notice of an asserted claim, the insurance carrier and physicians' attorney should be notified immediately, and copies of the lawsuit papers should be forward to each. It is imperative for the physician's attorney to know the exact circumstances under which the complaint was received, to whom it was delivered, who signed for receipt of the complaint, and the exact date and time of such receipt.

A medical malpractice complaint is difficult reading for the defendant physician, as the allegations frequently include punitive language that is often insulting. The named defendant must maintain emotional composure when reviewing the allegations of the complaint point by point and preparing to discuss them with counsel. Remember that the complaint purposely presents only one side of the story—it's biased. The complaint often includes language such as *willfully*, *wantonly*, and *recklessly* sprinkled throughout. The defendant will have an opportunity to respond in a factual matter, attempting to accurately depict the circumstances surrounding the allegations.

Upon notice of the malpractice claim, it is prudent for the defendant physician to transfer the care of the plaintiff to the care of another physician with similar training and expertise. After transfer to another physician, the defendant physician should have no contact or communication with the plaintiff, or legal representative for the plaintiff, except to provide copies of medical records to the patient or patient's designated representative as formally requested. All copies of records should be sent by certified mail. The physician should prevent any loss of or tampering with medical records.

Coverage Issues

When the malpractice insurer decides not to resolve the claim, control of the case will shift from the insurance company to the attorney retained to serve as independent counsel for the defendant physician. Defense counsel will be the physician's primary source for pertinent law and the progress of the case. The issues regarding the claim of negligence are directed to the defense counsel, and the attorney has a duty to keep the physician and insurance carrier informed about the progress of the case. The physician must be certain his or her counsel has no conflict of interest.

A professional liability insurance policy requires the company to provide a defense for the insured physician on all claims for which there may be potential coverage. If there is uncertainty surrounding a potential coverage issue, the carrier will issue a "reservation of rights" letter informing the physician that the company is providing defense counsel for the insured, but is reserving its rights to deny any coverage for any adverse settlements should the facts identified in the litigation support a denial. Among other reasons, the insurance company may deny coverage because some, or all of the treatment, occurred outside the coverage period, or the physician was treating outside his or her specialty, did not give proper notice when the claim arose, or had defaulted on payment and premiums. A physician should retain separate counsel to review any reservation of rights by the insurer, to provide advice about rights and obligations under the policy, and if necessary, to litigate against the insurance company in the event of wrongful dismissal of coverage.

MEETING WITH DEFENSE COUNSEL

Physician's Overview of the Case

Defense counsel will meet with the physician in person to find out about the particular facts underlying the claim, provide an overview of legal standards and issues that will be controlling, and discuss upcoming events in the case. The physician should arrange for the attorney to have all pertinent medical records, bills, devices, and instruments used that are pertinent to the claim, and a listing of all medical personal involved in the evaluation and treatment of the patient.

The physician must be prepared to describe in detail the diagnosis and treatment of the plaintiff, identify what personnel handled which aspects of treatment, and explain all notes and abbreviations in the medical records. The physician must familiarize the attorney with the normal causes, symptoms, and progression of the disease at issue, and how the diagnosed disease in question is typically treated. The attorney must be well-educated about the condition and treatments in question.

The physician must be completely candid with the attorney. If defense counsel is assuming false information to be true, he or she is primed for exposure that will cost credibility with the judge or jury, and will certainly decrease the likelihood of winning the case, or settling it favorably. True facts are critical for the defense counsel to evaluate the case and construct a defense. The attorney-client privilege, whereby the attorney and attorney's staff are ethically bound not to reveal any confidential communications, exists to specifically promote such full disclosure and will be violated only in situations such as to prevent the commission of fraud, or a future crime.

Identification of Other Parties

The physician's initial interview with counsel will allow identification of parties named in the lawsuit, and their roles in diagnosis and treatment. Plaintiff attorneys look for as many potential sources of recovery as possible, thereby naming all involved medical personnel and the clinic, or hospital were medical care was rendered. The defense attorney needs to identify healthcare professionals, or institutions involved in the patient's care that already settled claims against them.

The individual institutions need to be nominally named in the lawsuit for purposes of allocations of fault. The physician named in the lawsuit may want to file a cross claim against other parties, or add new unnamed parties. In this scenario, the physician would allege that the other defendant(s) are solely responsible for the plaintiff's injury, or if the physician is found liable to the plaintiff, that the other defendants or cross claimants should be obligated to reimburse him or her for the damages he or she has to pay

Evaluation of Procedural Pretrial Defenses

One of the procedural defenses to be considered is invalid or improper service of process. That is why it is imperative for the physician's attorney to know the exact circumstances under which the complaint was received, to whom it was delivered, who signed for receipt of the complaint, and the exact date and time of such receipt. If the method or timing of service were improper, the defense attorney may file a motion to dismiss the suit. This decision depends on the gravity of the improper services and the demeanor of the judge who decides the motion. The remedy for an improperly served complaint may be granting of additional time to allow proper service. Generally, unless the improper service is grossly abnormal, the defense counsel will move to the merits of the case as a possible reason for dismissal.

A motion to dismiss may be filed if the claim was filed beyond the statute of limitations, or if the plaintiff failed to comply with procedural, or other statutory requirements. The statute of limitations on a medical malpractice action varies from state to state, ranging from two to four years. The statute of limitations sets the time limit for filing suit and the clock does not begin until the alleged harm/injury has manifested itself.

The statute of limitations may be temporarily longer for claims involving minors, foreign bodies left in a patient's body, or claims where the harm was not reasonably discoverable for some period of time based upon the facts. Some states operate by a statue of repose. This sets out the maximum amount of time within which a lawsuit can be filed; the time when harm/injury manifests is not relevant.

Some states have statutes that require a plaintiff to certify that a competent medical professional in the same area of medical/surgical expertise has reviewed the claim and would be willing to testify as to the breach of the standard of care before a lawsuit can be filed.

Procedural defenses may be litigated as pretrial motions to dismiss. A motion to dismiss asks the court to find that even if everything in the complaint is true, the defendant is not liable, and should not be required to defend the lawsuit as a matter of law. The defendant physician may have to sign an affidavit, or sworn declaration, describing the circumstances supporting a motion to dismiss. Each side has an opportunity to present its legal argument on such a motion, as legal briefs or oral arguments at a hearing, and the judge will issue an order with a ruling.

Evaluation of the Merits of the Case and Substantive Legal Defenses

Substantive legal issues in the malpractice arena will allege issues such as negligence, improper informed consent, or an intentional tort, such as battery (operating on wrong appendage/organ). The elements of medical negligence are simple. The plaintiff must establish that the physician breached the standard of care in his or her evaluation and/or treatment, and that such breach was the proximate cause of the patient's alleged injury. The plaintiff tries to establish that the physician did not act as a reasonable physician with similar training would have under similar circumstances, and that the physician's error or omission made the patient's condition worse, slowed recovery, or caused injury or death.

The plaintiff will have to present testimony by expert witnesses that the standard of care was breached. The expert practicing in the relevant field of expertise will testify about the optimal evaluation and/or treatment of the particular condition, and identify any deviation from the standard of care. Expert testimony must also establish that the alleged negligence proximately caused the injury or illness, pain, and suffering allegedly endured by the plaintiff.

Assuming the case does not settle, the defendant physician will have the opportunity to present both factual and expert testimony, including experts retained to testify that the defendant physician followed the pertinent standard of care under the circumstances. The issues of breach of the standard of care and proximate cause will often boil down to the dueling of the experts, and the outcomes will depend on which experts present the most knowledgeable, objective, and credible testimony.

The two most straightforward and frequently asserted defenses are that the defendant physician did not breach the standard of care and/or that any error that the defendant physician may have made was not the proximate cause of patient's injury or condition progressing, or failing to improve. The burden lies with the plaintiff to establish these elements. The defense must present evidence disproving either or both of these elements.

Other defenses can shield the defendant physician even when all elements of negligence are proven. Additional potential defenses are independent intervening negligence and contributing negligence, which requires proving that despite the defendant physician's negligence, a co-incident or subsequent negligent act or omission was the real cause of the plaintiff's continued illness, injury, or death.

Contributory and comparative negligence are defenses to liability, when it can be shown that the plaintiff failed to act with the care of a reasonable person, and in so doing caused or contributed to her death or injury. The patient's negligence may be a partial or complete defense to liability. Additionally, every state has enacted some form of a Good Samaritan law, which shields a medical professional from liability for negligence. In Florida, a statue codifies a form of charitable immunity that state healthcare providers who offer free medical care to indigents are completely immune from a lawsuit for negligence.

Evaluation of the Plaintiff's Claim and of the Defendant Exposure

Medical malpractice plaintiffs are permitted to seek reimbursement for economic damages, non-economic damages, and punitive damages. Economic damages include lost earnings and expenses for medical treatment incident to and necessitated by the alleged act of negligence. Noneconomic damages refer to pain and suffering. Punitive damages are additional sums of money awarded to deter intentional, malicious, or reckless behavior.

Past economic damages typically include the dollar amount spent for alleged negligent care, any remedial care, and lost wages from work. In cases where the degree and cost of future medical care or future lost earnings potential are involved, each side will rely on expert testimony to establish what type and level of future care the plaintiff will need, and the potential for future gainful employment. This may require expert testimony from an economist to assist the jury in determining the award. Noneconomic and punitive damages are much more of a wild card than economic damages.

Pretrial Discovery Procedures

Once the complaint has been filed and answered, any procedural pretrial motions resolved, and a litigation strategy mapped out, the pretrial discovery process begins. The time interval from the time of alleged negligence to commencement of a malpractice claim may be several years. The discovery process will usually consume the largest portion of time once the lawsuit is filed. It is in the discovery process that the lawsuit is frequently won or lost. The attorneys typically control the discovery process.

The court is involved to the extent necessary to set timetables for completion of discovery, or to resolve any disputes among the parties about the propriety of requests or the timeliness and completeness of responses. The trial judge has the ultimate determination of what evidence may be considered by the jury at the trial. The rules of civil procedure govern the discovery process and provide two methods to identify what evidence or expert opinions the adversaries plan to offer at trial: written requests for information and live testimony of witness at deposition.

Written Discovery

Written discovery requests include requests for admission, requests for documents, and interrogatories.

Requests for admission are statements of facts that the recipient is asked to admit or deny under oath. If the recipient of the request fails to respond, the statement is automatically admitted as true. The recipient is typically instructed to provide a full explanation of the factual basis for his or her denial of any particular request.

Requests for documents are the means by which the plaintiff obtains copies of the physician's notes, records, bills, test results, and imaging results. Conversely, the defense attorney may serve similar requests upon the plaintiff, asking for all of the records of treatment by other physicians before, during, and after the defendant physician's treatment. Additional requests can include opinion letters, reports prepared by plaintiff's expert witnesses, and evidence of payment of plaintiff's damages from other sources.

Interrogatories are written questions submitted to the parties to the lawsuit asking for general information regarding the case, including explanations of the defendant's view of the facts, lists of people believed to have knowledge of the facts of the case, and information regarding previous claims filed against the defendant and the previous claims filed by the plaintiff. The responding party must obtain interrogatories under oath and they may be used at trial as if live testimony.

The defense attorney will review all incoming written discovery requests and identify response deadlines. The defense attorney and defendant physician should draft the responses together. The attorney identifies any requests that will not lead to admissible evidence and will object in writing to such requests. If opposing counsel disagrees, he or she may file a motion asking the presiding judge to rule on whether information sought is discoverable.

The defendant physician will review the responses of the plaintiff to interrogatories to evaluate accuracy and credibility and to identify any medical or factual mistakes and information omitted or unaccounted for. The defendant physician must review the reports of plaintiff experts to facilitate the defendant attorney's understanding as he or she prepares to depose the plaintiff's expert witnesses.

Depositions

A deposition is a witness's recorded testimony, given under oath, when questioned by the attorneys for the parties in the case. The deposition allows the attorney to find out what facts and opinions the witness will testify to at trial. The plaintiff attorney takes the deposition of the defendant physician, the physician's expert witnesses, and any fact witnesses the physician has identified. The defense attorney will take the depositions for the plaintiff and plaintiff witnesses. If the witness is one of the parties to the lawsuit, his or her attorney will be present to object to any allegedly improper questions, learn how his or her own witness presents, and ask follow up questions to clarify the witnesses answers or any misimpressions created on the record.

The attorney uses the deposition to lock down the witness's testimony to keep it from changing, to identify and explore any weaknesses, and to assess the witness's overall credibility and jury appeal. The strength or weakness of a witness or expert's deposition testimony is a crucial factor in a party's decision to settle the case or press forward to trial.

A witness physician must thoroughly prepare for deposition by having an in-depth knowledge of the patient's medical history and treatment. The plaintiff's attorney will use lack of in-depth knowledge to imply carelessness, callousness, indifference, and ignorance of the defendant physician. The defendant physician counsel will help the witness prepare for the deposition by telling him or her what to expect and by identifying possible questions the opposing counsel will ask.

Dispositive Motions

Upon completion of discover, either or both parties may file a motion for summary judgment, asking the court to rule in favor as a matter of law, even if the opposition's vision of the facts is considered to be true for purposes of the motion. The party moving for summary judgment must prove there is no genuine issues of material fact and therefore no need to proceed to trial. The moving party will file discovery depositions, transcripts, and legal briefs outlining his or her argument. Once the moving party has met its burden, the nonmoving party must file its own brief demonstrating a genuine issue for trial.

When the court considers summary judgment, it must view the undisputed facts and the inferences drawn from those facts in a light most favorable to the party opposing the motion for summary judgment. It is rarely granted in medical negligence cases because of the many factual issues and conflicting expert opinions.

Alternative Dispute Resolution/Mediation

Increasingly, courts encourage resolving disputes by agreement rather than trial. The judge may conduct a settlement conference or appoint a neutral third party to be a mediator or arbitrator of the dispute. The most common form of dispute resolution in medical malpractice cases is mediation.

At the mediation, all parties to the lawsuit, attorneys, and representatives from insurance companies meet in person with a neutral third-party mediator appointed by the court, or agreed upon by the disputing parties. The mediator does not decide the case, but attempts to get the parties to agree to settle on mutually agreeable terms. An excellent mediator will bring the parties together for an open, honest discussion about the merits of the case. The physician's demeanor will communicate to the plaintiff whether he or she is genuinely concerned for the plaintiff's well-being. What the physician says and how it is communicated will greatly affect whether a favorable agreement can be reached.

The mediation session offers each party an opportunity to speak with impunity. The statements made in the course of the mediation are privileged and may not be used by either party if the case proceeds to trial. It is an opportunity for the defendant's physician to express that he or she is sincerely sorry about the outcome.

The mediation will conclude when an agreement is reached or the communications come to an impasse. In a typical settlement agreement the parties will agree that the physician's settlement of the claim does not constitute an admission of liability, and the terms of the agreement are kept confidential. A physician should go into mediation with an open mind and willingness to explore all avenues of a peaceful resolution.

TRIAL

The trial begins with selection of a jury. A large pool of potential jurors will be questioned together and individually by the attorneys for each side about the potential juror's background, work experience, jury experience, and prejudices that may impair their ability to render a fair decision. Once the final composition of the jury is determined, the jurors will be sworn in and presentation of the case will begin.

In a medical liability case, the plaintiff carries the burden of proof, which in a civil trial requires establishing the elements of the case by a preponderance of the evidence. Thus, the burden is on the plaintiff to present evidence and persuade the jury. The defendant bears the burden of proof in affirmative defenses, such as whether the plaintiffs acted to cause or contribute to the injury.

Plaintiff counsel will call the plaintiff's witnesses and direct questions to elicit their direct testimony. Defense counsel will cross exam each witness, attempting to undermine credibility, demonstrate bias, or point out facts the witness did not acknowledge in testimony.

Once the plaintiff has finished presenting witnesses and evidence, the judge will entertain any motions by the defense for a direct verdict. This motion asks the judge to rule that the plaintiff has not provided sufficient evidence to allow the case to go to jury. Again, it is rare circumstance that this motion is granted.

Then the defense attorney will begin to present his or her evidence, including testimony of the defendant physician and supporting experts. The plaintiff's attorney will have an opportunity for cross-examination of the defendant physician and supportive experts. The defendant physician must remain composed when the plaintiff attorney attempts to discredit the physician during cross-examination. The attorneys will object to the admission of certain testimony or pieces of evidence as appropriate, and the judge will sustain or overrule this objection on the spot. At the conclusion of the defendant's presentation of evidence, the defendant may then again request the judge to decide the case based upon the law and not submit to the jury.

If the case moves forward, the attorneys conduct a conference during which they discuss and argue the elements of the instructions to the jurors. Then each attorney presents a closing argument to the jury. The judge will instruct the jury as to applicable law to the case, and how they are to deliberate and arrive at a verdict. Then the jury retires to deliberate. The foreman will announce verdict or impasse (hung jury). If a hung jury, the case may need to be retried.

POST-TRIAL MOTIONS AND APPEALS

Following the jury trial the losing side may move that the judge enter judgment notwithstanding the verdict. The threshold for this motion to succeed is extremely high, as the party so moving must establish no reasonable juror could have found in favor of the moving party based upon the evidence in the record. The losing side has a statutorily defined time period in which to file notice of its intention to appeal the verdict. The parties may settle before appeal.

CHAPTER 17

Are Doctors, PAs, and NPs at a Liability Risk?

T he demand for healthcare services continues to increase with the aging population and the influx of newly insured individuals under the Patient Protection and Affordable Care Act. The additional demand is presumed to exceed the capacity limits of the traditional physician-centric model of primary and subspecialty care. One response to meeting this increased demand has been the introduction of non-physician clinicians (NPCs)—physician assistants and nurse practitioners—into the healthcare system. Healthcare strategists believe this new practice model will help meet patient demands, decrease overall healthcare costs, and increase practice productivity.

This new paradigm may also add a complex level of responsibility and risk/liability often not recognized by the supervising physician. This is particularly true given the absence of a definite legal framework identifying how the co-employee relationship will affect the assignment of liability when negligence occurs.

Litigation against physicians and NPCs is increasing. Claim settlements are in the millions of dollars in the aggregate for PAs and NPs. The most common form of malpractice action against a healthcare provider, physician, or NPC is the tort of negligence. A tort is defined as a civil wrong for which there is a remedy in the form of damages. The plaintiff's attorney must prove four elements to be successful in a medical negligence lawsuit: 1) the physician has a duty of care to the individual; 2) the duty was breached by treatment that fell below the threshold to meet the standard of care; 3) the physician omission/commission was the proximate cause of the alleged harm; and 4) the plaintiff suffers compensable damages. Expert testimony is needed to establish the standard of care, breach of that standard, and that the negligence is the cause of the injury.

CLAIMS AGAINST PHYSICIANS FOR NPC MEDICAL ERRORS

The claims against physicians for NPC negligence in the traditional employer-employee relationship are well described in the literature. These claims are a foundation to understanding the responsibility of physicians working in concert with NPCs.

Alleged malpractice claims against physicians for errors of NPCs include:

- Lack of adequate supervision by the physician,
- Tardy or absent referral to a subspecialty care,
- Incorrect diagnosis or failure to identify the correct diagnosis,
- Physical examination/evaluation that is cursory or not performed,
- Misrepresentation of the credentials of the clinician, and
- Lack of due diligence in hiring the NPC.

These claims all fall within the "rubric of negligent-supervision" used to hold "masters" liable for the wrongful acts of "servants"

Cursory or absent supervision: When an NPC has limited or absent supervision (or limited or absent documentation of supervision) by a physician, the risk for allegations of negligent practice surfaces. Absent specific statutory or regulatory requirements, the question of appropriate supervision is a question of fact that is decided by the jury. Thus, practice context may be vital to a determination of the appropriateness of the supervision.

One physician supervising multiple NPCs increases the potential for a determination of inadequate supervision. One court found insufficient supervision by a physician who did not investigate a report by a patient that the care received from a PA was inappropriate. The facts determined that the PA-patient interaction was inappropriate and the physician was held liable for the actions of the PA under the theory of substandard supervision.

Tardy in time or absent referral to a more sophisticated level of care: An allegation of failure to properly diagnose/manage may be made when the NPC misinterprets the clinical history provided by the patient, resulting in a flawed or absent diagnose, and/or when attempts to treat a complicated medical/surgical illness are beyond the NPC's level of training and skill.

A pertinent example of an alleged malpractice claim based on failure to diagnose and tardy referral involved a patient treated at a U.S. Air Force base medical facility for months for a hiatal hernia with reflux. The plaintiff, a woman in her early 30s, had undergone medical care between 1980 and 1989 for diverse medical reasons. Because the medical care history resembles many of the complex patient scenarios confronted by medical providers, it is instructional to examine the facts. Below is a summary of the court's accounting of the plaintiff's medical care for the relevant period at a U.S. Air Force medical facility:

- **June 4, 1988**—The plaintiff was evaluated by a physician when presenting with vomiting, diarrhea, and hip pain. The physician diagnosed the plaintiff with chronic nausea.
- **June 17, 1988**—The plaintiff visited the PA complaining of pain in her hip and side, and continued pain in the area of her hiatal hernia. The PA diagnosed dyspepsia and prescribed Mylanta, Tagamet, and Motrin.
- **September 8, 1988**—The plaintiff complained of stomach bloating and heart burn to the PA. The PA diagnosed hiatal hernia with reflux. The PA prescribed Tagamet, Reglan, and Mylanta. The plaintiff's hip complaint was reviewed with the supervising physician. A CT scan and X-rays were ordered.
- **October 7, 1988**—The plaintiff saw the same PA for follow-up of her stomach and hip complaints. An upper GI revealed reflux and probable duodenitis. The PA continued the prescription for medication and prescribed a follow-up with the physician for hip pain.
- **October 12, 1988**—The plaintiff saw the physician for evaluation of her hip pain.
- **January 29, 1989**—At 8 a.m. the plaintiff awoke with severe upper abdominal pain. The plaintiff visited the emergency room with "crunching" pain in her upper abdomen and radiating up into her neck and down both arms. A GI cocktail did not alleviate her symptoms. A physician ordered an abdominal X-ray series. The physician reviewed the X-rays and diagnosed constipation and gave the patient a laxative. The physician recommended discharge but the plaintiff refused because she was in too much pain to go home. After further examination, an ECG was

ordered and revealed an evolving myocardial infarction. The treatment for the plaintiff's condition was not available and the attempt at transfer to a hospital was delayed in time. Upon arrival at the hospital, despite the referring physician's diagnosis of evolving myocardial infarction, the hospital physician initially treated the plaintiff for a hiatal hernia.

The plaintiff alleged medical negligence against the PA and physician and sought recovery from the defendants' employer, the United States. Based on the plaintiff's expert testimony, the court concluded, among other things, that the PA had substituted his judgment for that of a physician and that the physician was negligent for lack of supervision of the PA performance throughout the series of earlier appointments for multiple complaints.

Misrepresentation: Misrepresentation occurs when the patient is not informed that the NPC is not a physician. In one case, the jury found liability on this theory when a NPC prescribed a medication that resulted in an anaphylactic reaction leading to multi-organ system failure. The plaintiff alleged she was unaware she had been treated by a PA. She was not told when scheduling her appointment she would be seen by a PA and she was not corrected when she introduced the PA to her husband as "doctor." She claimed not to have noticed his name badge, business card, and signs inside and outside of the office identifying him as a PA.

Negligent hiring: Physicians and/or employers have a duty to use "due diligence" when hiring NPCs. Due diligence requires verification of educational background, licensure, and clinical experience. One court revoked a physician's license for "aiding and abetting" the unauthorized practice of medicine when they found he had not met the due diligence required when hiring a NPC. The physician had hired the PA based on the individual's attestation and did not independently verify the credentials.

LEGAL THEORIES

The legal underpinnings for the above-described malpractice allegations arise from three legal theories: 1) vicarious liability, 2) negligent supervision, and 3) negligent hiring. The legal theories are the conceptual framework used by the judicial review process to determine negligence/liability.

Vicarious liability imposes liability for a medical error by the wrongdoer (here, the NPC) to the principal (physician), the person on whose behalf the wrongdoer acted. The law of agency assigns vicarious liability under the respondeat superior and borrowed servant notions. The principal-agent relationship intrinsic to a vicarious liability claim under the theory of respondeat superior requires both that the master have the right to control the servant and that both parties voluntarily consent to the agent acting on behalf of the master. The Restatement (Second) Agency states that the master must have the right to voluntarily choose—to select and dismiss- the alleged servant.

Throughout the nation, the courts' interpretation of agency law as applied to physician–NPC relationships is mixed. An Alabama court in 2006, reviewing an alleged imputed claim of negligence, found that when there was no voluntary consent for a co-employee, nurse anesthetist, to work on behalf of the co-employee, anesthesiologist, there was no vicarious liability. Thus, the anesthesiologist would not be held liable.

A Wisconsin court reached the contrary conclusion in 2009 when it found a surgeon could be vicariously liable for a non-employee PA under the theory of respondeat superior. The court stated that respondeat superior, while typically arising in an employer-employee relationship, is not limited to only those situations.

In the Wisconsin case, an orthopedic surgeon performed hip surgery on the plaintiff's severely arthritic hip. A PA assisted the surgeon during surgery. Post-operation, the plaintiff had a new paralysis of the foot. The allegation was that negligent surgery resulted in the paralysis. The standard of care issue revolved around whether the paralysis resulted from the sciatic nerve or the peroneal nerve, which is a branch of the sciatic nerve. Sciatic nerve injury was a known potential complication and would not constitute a deviation from the standard of care.

The Appeals Court held that the surgeon's supervising role, required by the Wisconsin Administrative Code, might have been enough to conclude that the PA was acting under the physician's control and supervision even though there was no employer-employee relationship. The appellate court remanded the case to the trial court to determine if the facts supported a finding of the required control by the anesthesiologist over the PA for an imposition of vicarious liability.

In this case, the fact that there was no employer-employee relationship did not dispose of the potential for a finding of vicarious liability on the physician for the actions of the PA. The new corporate business medicine model alters the relationship between the NPC and physician: under the corporate model, both are employees of the corporate organization. This Wisconsin appellate court decision suggests that in some states the assignment of liability will be with the physician, who is presumed to control the actions of the NPC despite the absence of an employer-employee relationship. The Alabama court reached a polar-opposite conclusion.

The second legal underpinning for assignment of liability when physicians are working with NPCs is negligent supervision. This applies when the NCP performs clinical duties under the direction/supervision of the physician. Statutory law in certain states requires direct supervision and may determine whether the physician must be in the same location as the NPC. Physicians must strictly adhere to the statutory provisions to limit risk.

The third legal underpinning for assignment of liability is negligent hiring. This occurs when a physician hires a NPC, failing to use reasonable care to discover the NPCs lack of competence to perform the duties included in the clinical work.

NPCS WORKING WITH PHYSICIANS

Although the potential liability for actions of a NP in a retail clinic setting has been reviewed, there is no review of NP/PA liability when physicians are working with NPs in clinic and hospital settings and limited judicial decisions on this topic. Although most states require physician supervision and collaboration with NPCs, in some states, NPs have the ability to diagnose, treat, and manage patients independently of physicians.

Collaboration and supervising statutory schemes vary from state to state. The traditional requirement is that the NP work in connection with a physician to develop defined, written protocols under which the NP practices. Typically, the NP and the physician must spend onsite time together and have chart review requirements. These regulations appear to create a master-servant relationship, which, as articulated in the Restatement (Second) of Agency, could be subject to vicarious liability under respondent superior.

POLICY ISSUES

The dominant paradigm is that both the NPC and physician are co-employees of the corporate enterprise. It is the corporate entity, not the physician, which likely is imposing certain controls over what and how NPCs can perform and which patients they see. It is the employing entity that has control over which individuals are hired, retained and assigned to work together.

The present-day policy is focusing on improving efficiency and finances through the use of NPC in the delivery of care. This is an admirable goal, but possibly at a cost of providing less-sophisticated care. In making the decision to accept this sacrifice in exchange for efficiency and cost savings, policymakers will have to entertain the question as to who bears the liability when medical errors are made by the NPC. In addition to the negligent NPC, should the co-employee, supervising physician be vicariously liable?

A major goal of the tort law system is to limit the likelihood that similar errors of omission or commission will recur in the future. Shifting risk away from the NP and toward the supervising physician may hamper that goal. Eliminating the vicarious liability of the physician in this circumstance makes sense when the employing entity will likely provide the "deep pocket" for any uncompensated recovery from the negligent NPC.

CONCLUSION AND GOLDEN RULES

Physicians and NPCs working as co-employees of the corporate enterprise are navigating uncharted waters. Physicians would be prudent to be aware of the risks associated with a supervisory role over NPCs. Initially, physicians must realize they may be unwittingly assuming this liability risk. They should assume that a judicial review would identify the physician as having control of NPC's actions, even though the physician does not employ the NPC. Accordingly, the following are some golden rules for physicians:

- Become familiar and knowledgeable with the state rules, regulations, and requirements for the NPC in the state in which you practice.
- Affirm that the NPCs you work with meet all educational requirements and possess the experience and training needed to fulfill the position, including checking all credentials and references to ensure accuracy and veracity.

- Make efforts to properly teach, train, and monitor the NPC in areas of responsibility to ensure high-quality, safe patient care.
- Ensure that the ratio of physician-NPCs is commensurate with the number prescribed by law.
- Through the development of a system of high standards for NPCs, including regular review of patient management, focus on proper diagnosis, treatment, surveillance, and comprehensive mechanisms and documentation to ensure these standards are met.
- Lastly, when working as co-employees with NPCs, insert language in you contract indemnifying yourself and holding yourself harmless for liability that may be imposed for the negligence of the NPCs.

The physician performing these due diligence actions will minimize the risk for liability when working in conjunction with NPCs. It is imperative that you, the physician, understand the risks you assume in this new corporate medical world. The shift of risk in your direction must be met with unified resistance.

CHAPTER 18

The Intersection of Medical Education, Patient Care, and Law

Physicians in training (i.e., interns/residents, fellows) and advanced practitioners (nurse practitioners and physician assistants) are employed by the institution that sponsors their medical training program. The institution may be a community hospital or, more commonly, a hospital affiliated with an academic center. Due to varying levels of medical qualifications, physicians in training and advanced practitioners work under the supervision of attending physicians in a hierarchical fashion. The attending physicians are employees of the institution, or have a contractual relationship to teach the physicians in training.

Under common law, the employer has the right to dictate to the employee what to do as well as where, when, and how to do their assigned work. This type of strict employee-employer relationship typically exists between the training program and the healthcare trainee. In exchange, the institution or training program must provide to its employee continuing medical education, an environment where responsible patient care can be practiced, and protection against the medicolegal system during this critical learning period. It is this interwoven relationship that the physician in training, advanced practitioner, attending physician, and sponsoring institution of the graduate medical education are all at risk for allegations of negligence and potential defendants in a lawsuit.

INTERSECTION OF MEDICINE AND LAW

Physicians in training and advanced practitioners must be licensed to practice medicine and are subject to personal medical malpractice risk for providing care that does not meet the identified standard of care in the medical community. Physicians in training and nurse practitioners must recognize the impact of the law in graduate medical education. The greatest concern for training physicians and physician extenders is the potential for personal encounters with the law. The Accreditation Council for Graduate Medical Education (ACGME) requires accredited institutions that sponsor residency and fellowship programs to provide professional liability insurance. Examples that demonstrate the sometimes tortuous relationship between medical education and the law include the antitrust lawsuit against the Association of American Medical Colleges, the federal regulation of resident work hours, Medicare and Medicaid ever changing compliance regulations, the complexities of the Health Insurance Portability and Accountability Act of 1996, and the growing concern with the legal ramifications of the electronic medical record and the exponential growth in rules and regulations associated with guideline and metric medicine.

The attending physicians and sponsoring institutions are aware of, and concerned about, the potential for professional liability. The complex relationship between physician trainees, nurse practitioners, attending physicians and sponsoring institutions make the legal issues an important topic for discussion. In the future, graduate medical education will continue to be constrained by current and evolving rules of law.

THE STANDARD OF CARE

Healthcare providers and graduate medical education institutions together share a responsibility to provide high-quality and safe patient care in accordance with standards of care established in medicine. The law has not, and will not, proffer a lower threshold for meeting the standard of care for physicians in training or advanced practitioners. Physicians in training are held to the same standard of care as attending physicians. This principle encourages physicians in training to seek supervision and inspires attending physicians to provide close, vigilant oversight.

Attending physicians are exposed to malpractice allegations for the care they provide directly and indirectly through their supervision of physicians in training. Attending physicians may be held vicariously liable for the negligence of physician in training under their supervision and directly liable for insufficient supervision. The adequacy of supervision is continually being elevated to higher standards as the public's attention to patient safety continues to escalate. The graduate medical education institutions and program sponsors bear legal responsibility for the care they deliver and the negligence of their employees. They also face liability for failure to administer safe systems of care. Physicians in training, advanced practitioners, attending physicians, and graduate medical education organizations all must understand and meet these substantial legal standards.

PHYSICIANS IN TRAINING STANDARD OF CARE

What standard of care should apply to a physician in training? Courts have held that trainees should be held to the same standard of care as attending physicians. Courts walk a slippery slope when determining where to hold trainees accountable using an objective, equitable standard of care that facilitates the essential educational mission of training, yet assures for patient safety, and an opportunity for patients to seek redress for their injuries. Modern jurisprudence favors holding the trainee/advanced practitioner/attending triad to the standard of care of an attending in that particular specialty. This is a reasonable and sensible standard given the education and training process is dependent upon the attending physician's teaching and supervisory role.

The rationale for insisting on this standard for training physicians is grounded in a public policy that protects the safety of patients. Courts have noted a benevolent dual purpose: 1) creating an incentive for physicians in training to seek supervision, and 2) incentivizing attending physicians to provide the highest quality supervision. Physicians in training should expect to be held to the same standard of medical care as a reasonable attending physician in their specialty based upon the precedent of the available case law.

Graduate medical education institutions must ensure risk management considerations bolstering patient safety by mandating training physicians seek attending physician advice whether certain or uncertain about the patient's medical conditions. Attending physicians must be available to provide the supervision needed to provide the highest quality of care. The discussion between the trainee and the attending physicians has great value in evaluating the appropriateness of the trainee's thinking and plan of medical care.

In general, the Accreditation Council for Graduate Medical Education (ACGME) requires accredited institutions that sponsor residency and fellowship programs to provide professional liability insurance to cover all claims arising within the scope and duration of the training. This *occurrence-based* coverage provides for a legal defense and financial protection against claims connected to medical care implemented during a training physician's activities while a participating in a graduate medical education program. The ACGME standards do not mandate that the policies apply to medical practice outside the graduate medical education program. Sponsoring institutions must provide appropriate clinical support for trainee physicians in compliance with collaborative, supervisory agreements with attending physicians.

ADVANCED PRACTITIONERS' STANDARD OF CARE

Liability Issues

Physician assistants and nurse practitioners, or physician extenders, are considered legally liable for actions or omissions concerning patients they treat, and therefore, required in all states to carry adequate medical liability insurance.

Physicians providing medical direction and/or supervision may also be held liable for the actions or omissions of PAs and NPs, even if no patient/physician interaction occurred. Such liability exists in three separate manners: *negligent selection, negligent supervision, and respondent superior.*

The medical director and/or other party responsible for hiring a physician assistant or nurse practitioner may be accused of *negligent selection*, claiming that the party responsible for hiring the physician assistant or nurse practitioner knew, or should have known, prior issues in the physician assistant's or nurse practitioner's past that may have predicted future performance insufficiencies. Diligent research and reference review, with adequate documentation of same, should help prevent and protect from such claims.

Negligent supervision may be alleged against the supervising physician of record, claiming that the supervising physician did not follow state, hospital or departmental supervision regulation/policies/guidelines, or if the plaintiff's expert believes the physician's supervision was otherwise below the standard of care. In order to decrease ambiguity, emergency departments utilizing advanced practitioners should have guidelines specifying supervising physician responsibility, including factors that trigger when a physician assistant or nurse practitioner should seek supervising physician consultation, and when a supervising physician should physically attend to a patient evaluated by a physician extender.

If not named for any of the aforementioned reasons, a supervising physician may be included in a medical liability action against a physician extender under the *respondeat superior* claim. *Respondeat superior*, Latin for "let the master answer," is the primary vehicle used to assert vicarious liability of the supervising physician for the alleged negligent acts of physician extenders. Under this principle, the supervising physician may not have been present or even aware of the patient encounter, but as the "master of the ship" may be considered liable. Should no claim of negligent selection or supervision be raised, often, supervising physicians named under the concept of *respondeat superior* will eventually be dismissed from the case.

Historically, there have been fewer medical liability cases brought against physician extenders. In 2009, Hooker, Nicholson, and colleagues undertook a 17-year review of the United States National Practitioner Data Bank from 1991 through 2007. During the study period, the probability of making a malpractice payment was 12 times less for physician assistants and 24 times less for nurse practitioners as compared to physicians.

ATTENDING PHYSICIANS STANDARD OF CARE

Attending physicians supervising training physicians in graduate medical education setting are subject to the same liability exposure they face when they personally direct and deliver care outside the graduate medical education arena. The attending physician's liability risk is unaffected by the nature of the relationship with the sponsor of the training program. Attending physicians are exposed to two additional types of liability when assuming a supervisory role: 1) vicarious liability for the physician in training's negligence under the respondeat superior notion, and 2) direct liability for failure to supervise. Courts focus on the nature and extent of the attending physician's control over the practice setting, and the control of the institution under which the training physician is working. Frequently, both the attending physician and the sponsoring institution may be vicariously liable.

PRESENT-DAY MEDICAL PRACTICE

These evolving and growing legal standards are juxtaposed to the fact that physicians working in hospitals are being asked to do more in less time—the impact of corporate medicine and the RVU as the metric of productivity. The arsenal of tests, technologies, and therapies are accelerating at an exponential rate. Concerns over neglectful medical decisions made under extreme fatigue have resulted in reduction of resident work hours. Consequently, this change in trainee working hours has led to an increasing number of "handoffs" of patients between changing shifts and continuity of care may be compromised. This change in the healthcare landscape has mandated that attending physicians and their extenders be more aware of the details of each patient's health status to better coordinate the care of patients being cared for by physicians in training.

Inpatient care at hospitals has become a relay race between training physicians, advanced practitioners, and attending physicians—the patient is the baton and coordination of the patient's care is a challenge. These changes have led to a more turbulent work environment. Medical care is susceptible to the level of emotional, biological, and physical resilience of attending physicians, nurse practitioners, and physicians in training. Physicians need an internal compass to cope with the changing landscape of medical care to preserve the sanctity of patient care. The large number of variables involved in patient care leaves us susceptible to medical errors and for potential allegation of negligence.

See Chapter 17 for a detailed discussion of lawsuits.

CHAPTER 19

Medical Staff
Peer Review

Medical peer review is the process by which a professional review body considers whether a practitioner's clinical privileges or membership in a professional society will be adversely affected by a physician's competence or professional conduct. The foremost objective of the medical peer review process is the promotion of the highest quality of medical care as well as patient safety.

The Health Care Quality Improvement Act of 1986 (HCQIA), sets out standards for professional review actions. If a professional review body meets these standards, then neither the professional review body nor any person acting as a member or staff to the body will be liable in damages under most federal or state laws with respect to the action.

The HCQIA requires that a professional review body provide adequate notice and a hearing to the physician involved. Pursuant to the HCQIA, an appropriate notice must include:

- A statement to the physician that a professional review action has been proposed to be taken against the physician;
- A statement to the physician the reasons for the action;
- An indication that the physician may request a hearing, and any applicable time limits for making the request; and
- A summary of the physician's rights in the hearing.

If a timely request for a hearing is made, the professional review body must provide the physician notice of the hearing, including a list of witnesses expected to testify on the professional review body's behalf. The hearing cannot be scheduled for less than 30 days after the date of the notice.

The HCQIA permits hearings to be held before an officer, panel or an arbitrator. At the hearing, the physician has the right to:

- Representation by an attorney, or any other person of the physician's choice;
- Call, examine, and cross examine witnesses;
- Present evidence;
- Submit a written statement at the conclusion of the hearing; and
- Have a record made of the proceedings.

After the hearing, HCQIA requires that the hearing officer, hearing panel, or arbitrator advise the physician involved of any recommendation(s) in writing. In the case of determining whether to grant, suspend, or revoke a physician's hospital staff privileges or medical staff membership, a hospital's governing body makes the ultimate determination. However, the recommendations of a peer review body strongly influence the governing body's decision.

In order to provide incentive for physicians and others to participate in medical peer review, federal and state law works to protect peer review participants and processes. In every state, some combination of the following statutory protections is available to good faith peer review:

- Involved individuals and institutions are granted immunity from lawsuits;
- Information related to the peer review process is deemed confidential; and
- Peer review work product is designated privileged and inadmissible in court.

The American Medical Association (AMA) supports the medical peer review process and recommends that peer review evaluations should be based upon appropriateness, medical necessity, and efficiency of services in order to assure quality medical care. The AMA advises that any system of medical peer review should have established procedures. Furthermore, the AMA advocates that the peer review process should protect the confidentiality of medical information obtained and used in conducting peer review.

Federal law related to Medicare and Medicaid programs mandate some form of peer review if hospitals are to be compensated for services, and the

Joint Committee on Accreditation of Healthcare Organizations (JCAHO) also requires its member hospitals to have a credentialing process in place for accreditation. Therefore federal and state law, regulations, and professional organizations all emphasize a hospital's duty to monitor patient care and serve as the impetus for credentialing.

The HCQIA grants healthcare entities and peer review committees immunity from liability for credentialing and privileging activities as long as due process is afforded the affected physician. The critical issue is the appropriate application of due process. The HCQIA also established the National Practitioner Data Bank (NPDB), an information clearinghouse regarding licensure actions, malpractice payments, and final adverse actions taken by hospitals and other healthcare entities that restrict physicians' practice privileges for more than 30 days. Hospitals and other healthcare entities must also query the NPDB when credentialing physicians for appointment and reappointment to the medical staff.

CREDENTIALING

Case law regarding credentialing generally supports the premise that a hospital could be held liable for a patient injured by a staff physician because the hospital should have known of the physician's poor performance or incompetence and failed to investigate or take reasonable corrective action. A Wisconsin case, *Darling v. Charleston Community Memorial Hospital*, ruled that the hospital had a duty to properly credential physicians on its staff even when the physician falsified his or her application for privileges. Similarly, courts have held that the hospital may be responsible for the conduct of its physicians under the doctrine of corporate negligence. These cases underscore the need for ongoing peer review to maintain quality care.

All credentialing criteria, including appointments, standards and appeal rights, must be clearly stated in the medical staff bylaws and communicated to members of the medical staff and new applicants.

PRIVILEGING

The objective of the privileging decisions should be the delineation of the specific diagnostic and therapeutic procedures, whether medical or surgical, that may be performed in the hospital and the types of clinical situations to be managed by the physician. The JCAHO requires that privileges be granted before any care is provided to patients, noting that temporary privileges must be time limited. Physicians working in outpatient facilities owned or managed by JCAHO-approved health care entities are also subject to the credentialing and privileging process.

PROCTORING

Proctoring is a process of direct observation that allows for the focused evaluation of current physician cognitive and procedural competency. If the proctor observes potential or imminent patient harm during the proctoring process, it may be ethically appropriate for him or her to intervene. For all new applicants for privileges and for physicians who may be returning to practice, proctoring is usually required for a time to ensure that the physician is competent to perform the procedures for which privileges are requested. Appropriate proctors should be selected and can include members of the medical staff who are non-competitors, when possible, and senior active staff who have privileges in the same area of practice. As in other areas of credentialing and peer review, the reviewing body must follow principles of due process.

DUE PROCESS

The Supreme court has defined due process as (1) giving written notice of the actions contemplated, (2) convening a hearing, (3) allowing both sides to present evidence at the hearing, and (4) having an independent adjudication.

These principles of fair play apply in all disciplinary hearings and in any other type of hearing in which the reputation, professional status, or livelihood of the physician or medical student may be negatively impacted. They apply when the hearing body is a medical society tribunal, a medical staff committee, or another similar body composed of peers.

All physicians and medical students are urged to diligently observe these fundamental safeguards of due process whenever they are called upon to serve on a committee that will pass judgment on a peer. All medical societies and institutions are urged to review their constitutions and bylaws and/or policies to make sure that these instruments provide for such procedural safeguards. Clearly written due process procedures must be established, understood, and properly implemented by the hospital because physicians have legal rights to protect their careers. Prior to the Health Care Quality Improvement Act of 1986 (HCQIA), an adverse peer review finding remained with the reviewing hospital. Because the HCQIA mandates peer review committees to report disciplinary actions to the National Practitioner Data Bank, an adverse report now could harm a physician's prospects for employment throughout the nation.

APPLICATION OF DUE PROCESS PRINCIPLES

Due process requires that the right to practice medicine not be infringed upon in an arbitrary or capricious manner. The critical question concerns what procedures will suffice to satisfy due process requirements. Unfortunately there are no answers to this query; due process varies according to the facts and circumstances of each case and according to the law of each jurisdiction where it is applied.

Although the type of hearing afforded may vary from case to case, due process clearly requires some form of hearing before an individual may be deprived of a protected interest. Furthermore, it is generally accepted that in a highly technical occupation like the practice of medicine, the members of the profession should have the power to set their own standards, but the standards and evaluations must be made in good faith and protect against arbitrary and capricious actions. On the other hand, there is no constitutional requirement that physicians be given a formal adversarial hearing, nor even that the decision-makers be completely uninvolved in the underlying matter. The common law requirement of a fair procedure does not compel formal proceedings with all the embellishment of a court trial, nor adherence to a single mode of due process. It may be satisfied by any one of a variety of procedures that afford a fair opportunity for an applicant to present his position.

Although medical staff bylaws vary from one institution to the next, most are similar in providing for an initial investigation by a credentials committee or similar body, during which the physician generally has few procedural rights, but may be required to appear and answer questions in the matter; a hearing, including the basic elements previously discussed;

and an appeal to the governing board of the hospital, medical society, or other institution. Medical societies have promulgated model medical staff bylaws prescribing procedures for each of these steps, and these models are generally geared toward ensuring a fair procedure for the physician whose privileges are under review.

The final element of due process in adverse actions affecting staff privileges is that of judicial review. This right also varies considerably from one jurisdiction to another, again depending on each state's interpretation of due process, the property or liberty rights recognized, and the extent to which the courts have been willing to intervene in what have traditionally been considered private, or semipublic, concerns. Nevertheless, the majority of jurisdictions now recognize the right to obtain redress in the courts if the institution fails to provide due process, with respect to medical staff privileges. Judicial review may be limited to a review of the written record of proceedings held by the peer review body or may encompass a full evidentiary hearing de novo, although the latter may be available only under limited circumstances.

CONFIDENTIALITY AND PEER REVIEW PRIVILEGE

Generally, records of peer review actions and proceedings are exempted from discovery and evidentiary use in civil actions. Exceptions are sometimes found in cases in which a plaintiff has made a bona fide, prima facie case against the hospital for negligently credentialing the physician or in which the litigation concerns the physician's rights against the institution (as opposed to a malpractice claim).

Confidentiality may be ensured by means other than the law. Medical staff bylaws often require members involved in peer review proceedings to hold confidential all information and records relating to the proceedings or otherwise be subjected themselves to disciplinary action.

PEER REVIEW CORRECTIVE ACTION

Most physicians carry hospital staff privileges in one or more facilities. The medical staff is self-policing and is independent of the hospital. Its functions include reviewing the care provided by its physician members to patients and acting as a liaison between the hospital administration and individual physicians. As a peer review body, the medical staff is responsible for shielding patients from incompetent or unstable physicians; at the same time, by controlling physicians' access to both the patients and the facilities, the medical staff wields considerable power over physicians, and when that power is abused, the physician's professional reputation, standing, and license to practice may be disrupted and damaged.

Despite a growing trend toward protecting physicians' fundamental rights and interests in medical staff privileges, medical staffs continue to operate independently, without strict controls, when determining which physicians are granted credentials and which physicians should lose their credentials.

It is important to understand that at every stage of the disciplinary process, the affected physician is at a disadvantage. The disciplinary hearing under medical staff bylaws is like a malpractice action against the affected physician with one's own colleagues acting as witnesses, prosecutors, and judges. Charges involving the care of numerous patients may be leveled at one time. If the physician loses, he or she will probably have no insurance coverage for the defense costs of the disciplinary hearing or the economic impact on his or her medical practice.

There is little opportunity to obtain discovery of evidence before it is presented. The chairman of the medical executive committee usually selects the jury panel members and hearing officer. There may be use of hearsay evidence, including medical opinions of experts who cannot be compelled to appear and be cross-examined. Frequently, the physician is denied the assistance of counsel in the hearing room and must represent him or herself or depend on a medical colleague to act in a representative capacity. Other procedural protections, such as the right to subpoena witnesses or documents, are usually lacking, and witnesses in a peer review hearing may enjoy absolute immunity from civil suits for slander or malicious injury, even if their testimony is false. The hospital and medical staff members are also immune from suit under federal law unless it is proved that they acted in bad faith when taking the peer review action.

An adverse outcome for the physician may destroy his or her career. Actions adversely affecting medical staff privileges must be reported by the hospital to the state medical board, as well as the NPDB and the Healthcare Integrity and Protection Data Bank, nationwide data bases accessible to hospitals and managed care organizations. The state Medical Board may then commence an investigation, finding the physician an easy target because damning evidence has already been compiled in the medical staff hearing. Although the state medical board may decide not to prosecute, in almost all cases it can do nothing to aid the physician to clear his or her name, regain staff privileges, or obtain redress for the economic, professional, and emotional injuries sustained. The physician's reputation and career may be ruined, and his or her legal recourse is extremely limited. Although physicians have sued for deprivation of hospital staff privileges on any number of legal theories, including breach of contract, various tort theories, and antitrust, these suits are difficult, costly, and rarely successful.

Although the objective of peer review is to ensure the quality of care and retention of competence of medical staff, peer review functions as performed by physician staff members who are uncompensated for their efforts retain the risk of being sued by the affected physician despite immunity statutes. In addition, peer review immunity may not necessarily be extended if a federal claim, such as antitrust or unlawful discrimination, is proved.

LOSS OF PRIVILEGES UNRELATED TO PEER REVIEW

Numerous instances continue to exist in which a physician's medical staff privileges may be revoked or withdrawn and due process protections cannot be invoked, such as when a hospital acts for purely business or economic reasons or some other cause that does not relate to the quality of care practiced by the physician or his or her fitness to practice. For example, courts have held that a hospital may close its staff or a particular service, such as radiology or anesthesiology, or award an exclusive contract to one physician or group while excluding all others (including those already on staff). Although such actions have occasionally been challenged on both due process and antitrust theories, these cases have failed to produce decisions limiting the hospital's discretion to make such decisions, even when the resulting effects on individual physicians are harmful or seemingly anticompetitive.

www.ingramcontent.com/pod-product-compliance
Lightning Source LLC
Chambersburg PA
CBHW061314220326
41599CB00026B/4867